Contents

About Me

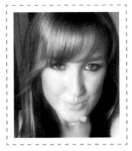

I'm Natalie wife and mother to my beautiful little girl Annabelle.

I have always had a passion for cooking but have been far too busy (lazy!) to ever take it seriously, however when I became a mother for the first time food suddenly became extremely important to me, I wanted to be as healthy as I could be during my pregnancy and at six months of age teach my daughter that she can fuel her body in a healthy yet exceptionally tasty way!

A local NCT course convinced me that baby led weaning is beyond doubt the best way to wean and once I got started I was amazed at how exciting Annabelle and I found it, I got the baking bug and starting trying every suitable recipe I could find, I then began adjusting recipes to improve them, make them naughtier for special occasions or healthier for every day consumption. I also had to make some simple adjustments to ingredients because Annabelle suffers with a cow milk allergy.

After spending hours on end tweaking recipes and writing them up in my little notebook I thought it would be a lovely idea to share them with other mums who would like to go the baby led weaning route and prove that other cows milk allergy suffers can have as much fun with food as any other BLW baby!

I hope you and your baby enjoy the recipes as much as Annabelle and I do!

Natalie x

About Baby Led Weaning

Baby Led Weaning is simply skipping past the puree stage of traditional weaning and offering your baby smaller portions of your own food from around the age of six months. Baby Led Weaning is focused on baby experiencing real tastes and textures from the very beginning of their weaning journey. This method also promotes family mealtimes and means the whole family can eat the same food together.

My goal is to supply you with recipes that are quick to prepare yet nutrient rich so baby can grow up enjoying healthy, nutritious but above all TASTY foods!

IMPORTANT: Before you start baby led weaning please consult your doctor to ensure this form of weaning is appropriate and safe for your child.

The Benefits:

- It gives your baby the opportunity to explore the taste, texture, color and smell of food
- It helps develop hand-eye coordination
- Establishes great eating habits as baby is allowed to eat as much as she/he needs, in their own time
- Your less likely to have a fussy eater
- Saves time not having to cook separate food for baby
- Promotes family mealtimes

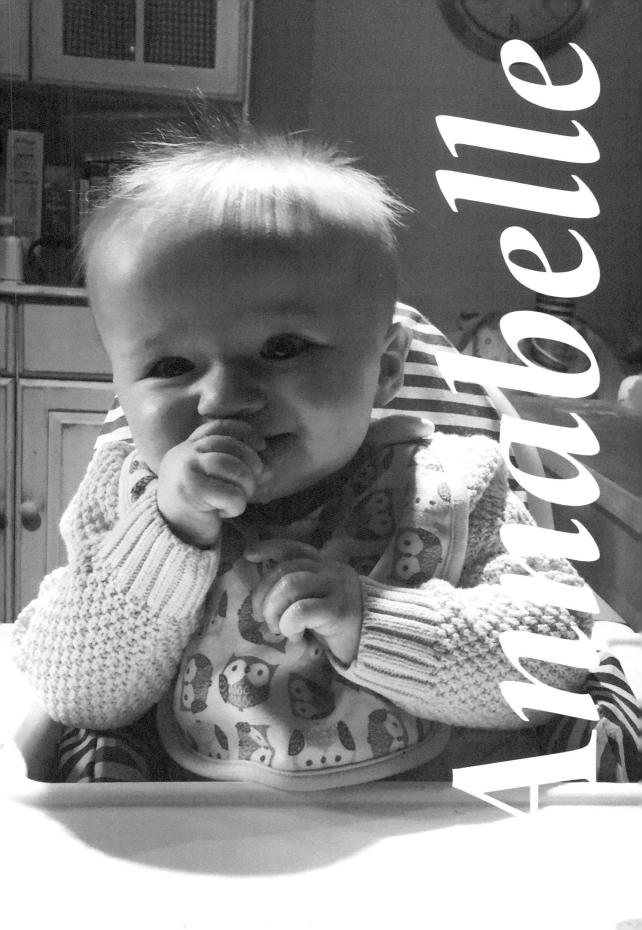

Annabelle

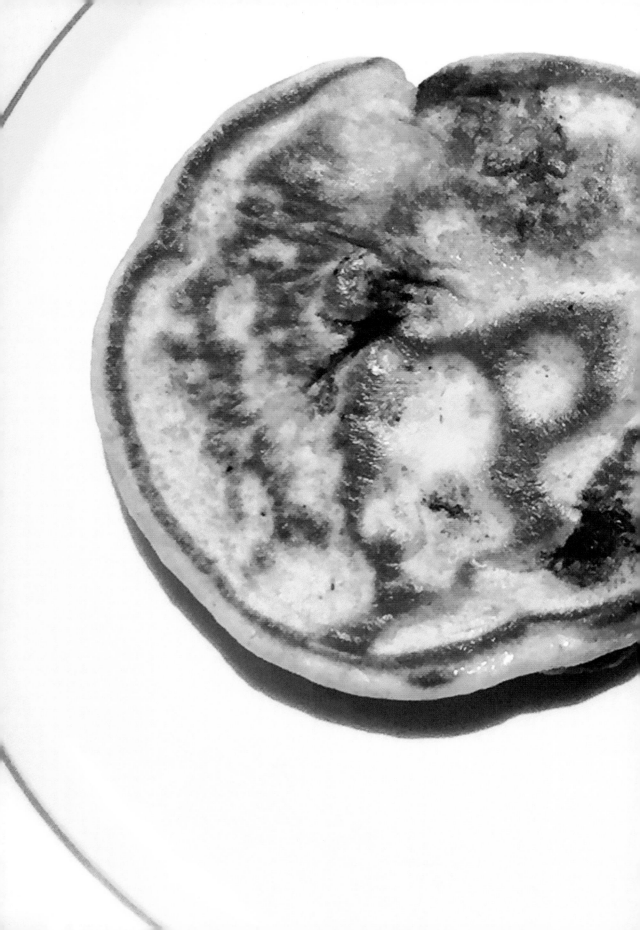

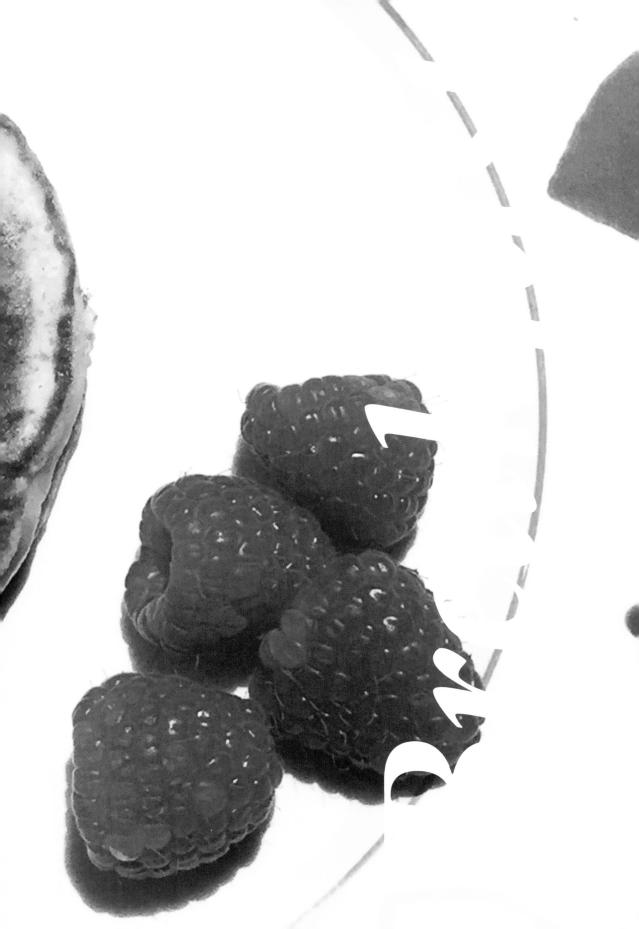

Banana Toast

This delicious and moist banana toast is perfect for baby led weaning beginners! It quick to prepare and its moist texture make it very easy for bub to munch.

- -

Prep Time: 5 mins
Cook Time: 4 mins
Yields: 2

- -

Ingredients

1 banana, mashed or blended till smooth
60ml milk (cows, soya, breast or formula)
Unsalted butter for frying
2 slices of bread

- -

Method

- Mix mashed banana and milk in a small bowl and then transfer onto a plate
- Soak each slice of bread in the mix for 1 minute on each side
- Heat butter in a pan and fry each slice of bread for 2 minutes on each side
- Serve in soldier style slices

Breakfast

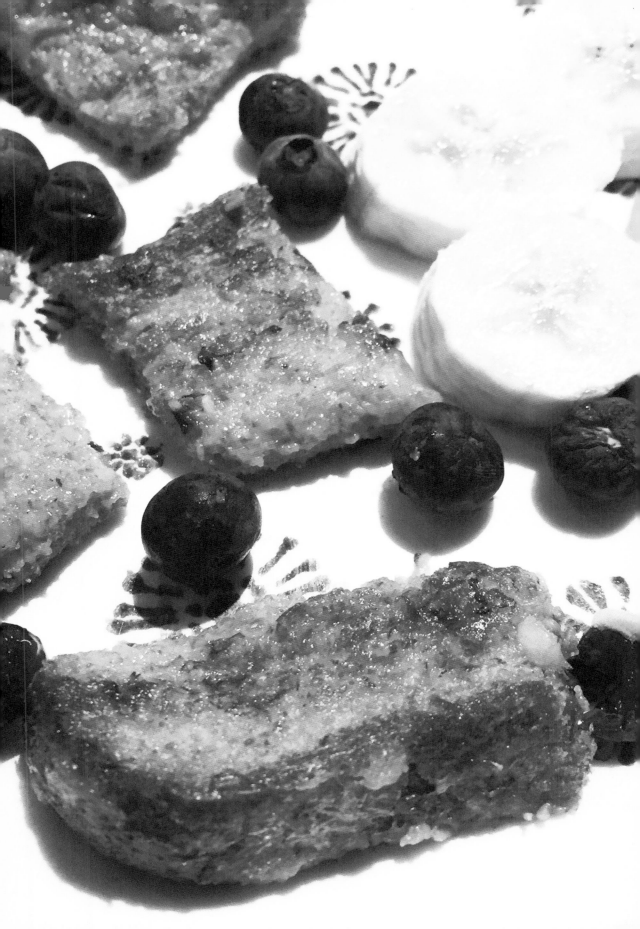

Maple French Toast

This maple French toast is so delicious that Annabelle and I could eat this for breakfast, lunch or dinner. Annabelle is very much a carb lover just like her mum so anything with bread or pasta in is guaranteed to be a hit!

- -

Prep Time: 5 mins
Cook Time: 3 mins
Yields: 3-4

- -

Ingredients

6 eggs
1 cup milk
1 tsp cinnamon
1 tsp vanilla bean paste, or extract
2 tbsp maple or agave syrup (plus extra to serve if you so desire)
6 slices of bread

- -

Method

- Mix all ingredients in a medium bowl
- Pour mix onto a plate and soak each slice of bread for 2 minutes on each side
- Heat oil in a frying pan over a medium heat and add eggy bread, fry each slice for 2-3 minutes on each side (until golden brown in color) - this will need to be done in batches
- Serve cooled with a selection of fruit

- -

Additional Info

Please feel free to half recipe if desired however leftovers can be frozen.

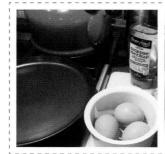 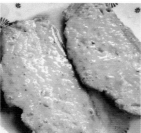 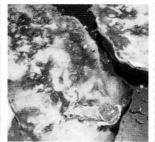

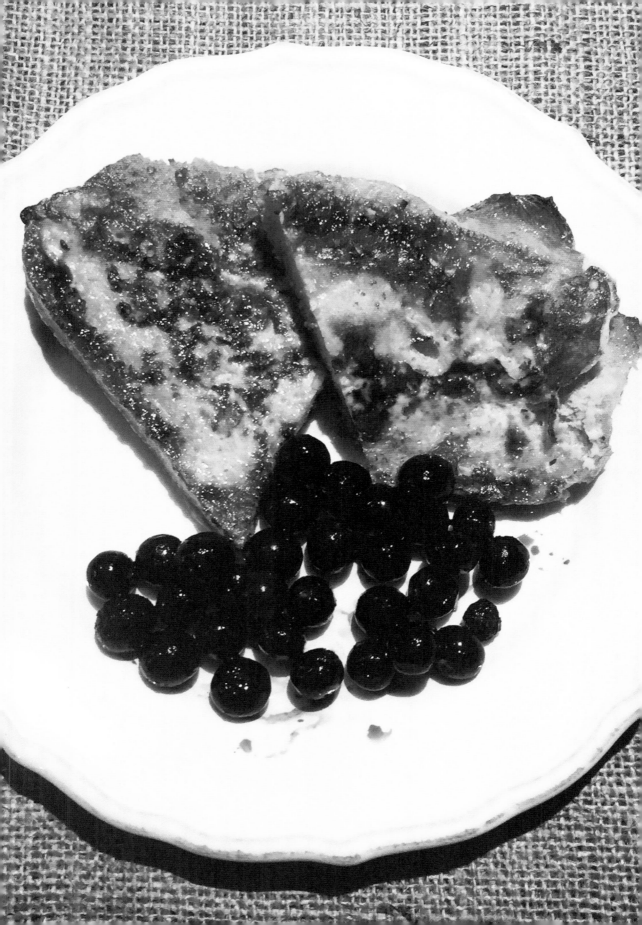

Mini Porridge Bakes

These are simply delicious – I love them especially because you can a create a batch with so many variable toppings your baby can have a different flavor every day of the week. They work well for breakfast or as a snack – they would also be lovely packed into a lunch box.

Prep Time: 15 mins
Cook Time: 35 mins
Yields: 24

Ingredients

Butter for greasing two muffin tins
2 eggs, whisked
2 mushed bananas
1 tbsp agave or maple syrup
2 1/2 cup old fashioned oats (cheap ones, not instant)
1 tbsp cinnamon
1 1/2 tsp baking powder
1 1/2 cup of milk (cows, soya, oat, coconut, hazelnut or almond)
1 tsp vanilla bean paste or extract

Method

- Heat oven to 180°C
- Grease 2 x 12 muffin tins
- Mix eggs, vanilla, bananas and agave in a large bowl
- In a smaller bowl mix oats, cinnamon and baking powder and then combine with banana mix
- Stir in your choice of milk
- Divide mix between 2 muffins tins
- Once filled top the mix with your choice of toppings, you could try: choc chips, strawberries, raspberries, blueberries, mango, granola

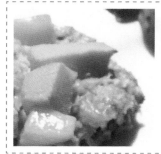 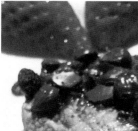 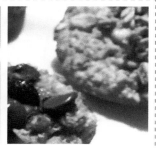

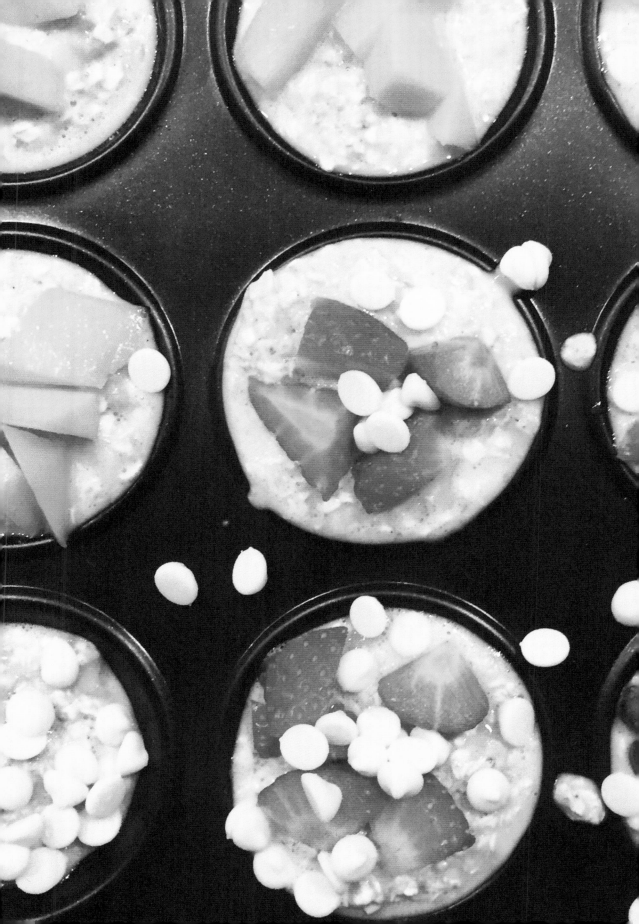

Mini Pancake Bites

These mini pancakes look and taste delicious – hopefully the prettiness of them will entice even the fussiest of eaters!

Prep Time: 15 mins
Cook Time: 15 mins
Yields: 24

Ingredients

1 1/2 cups plain flour
3 1/2 tsp baking powder
1 tbs sugar
2 tbsp of unsalted melted butter
1 1/4 cup milk
1 egg

Method

- Heat oven to 180°C
- Sift flour, baking powder and sugar into a large bowl - mix well
- Combine eggs, butter and milk in a separate bowl - whisk well
- Slowly pour the egg mix into the flour mix and whisk to create a smooth runny batter
- Pour batter into 2 x 12 muffin tins - filling each 3/4 full
- Once tins are filled you can top batter with ingredients of your choice
  - strawberries, raspberries, blueberries, chocolate chips, bacon and cheese, jam, raisins
- Once toppings have been added place trays in the oven for 15 - 20 mins or until starting to golden very slightly

---

Additional Info

For extra sweetness serve with maple or agave syrup.

Breakfast

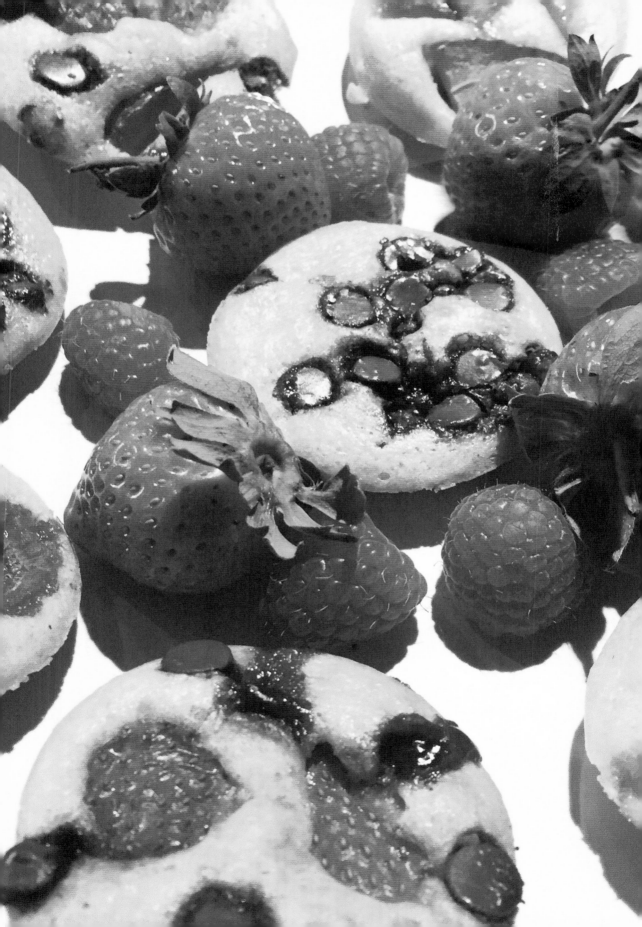

Blueberry Drop Scones

Prep Time: 10 mins
Cook Time: 4 mins
Yields: 10

Ingredients

1 cup self raising flour
1 egg
150ml milk (soya for cows milk allergy)
1 cup blueberries (fresh or frozen)

Method

- Add the flour to a large bowl - make a well in the middle and break egg into it
- Slowly add the milk - whisking until there are no lumps and you have a smooth thick batter
- Gently fold in the blueberries
- Heat oil in a pan and add 2 tablespoons of batter per scone - fry each scone for 2 minutes on each side

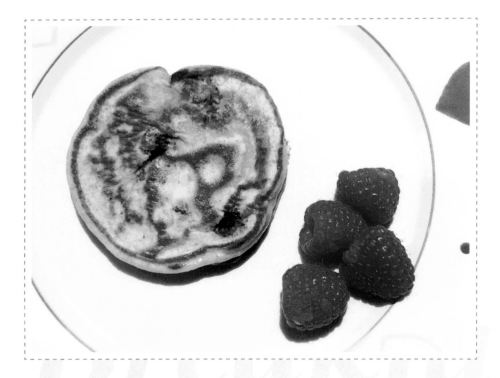

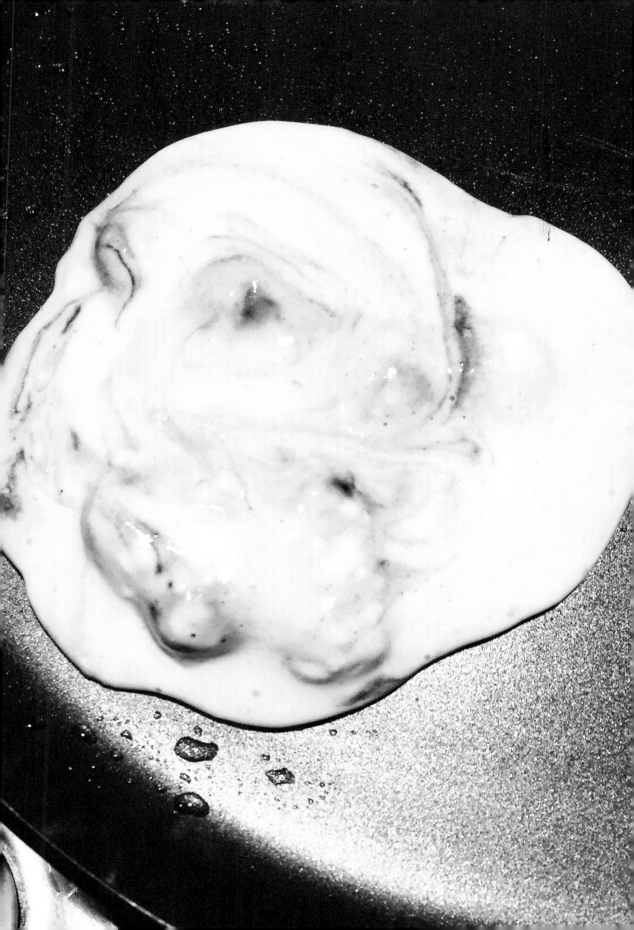

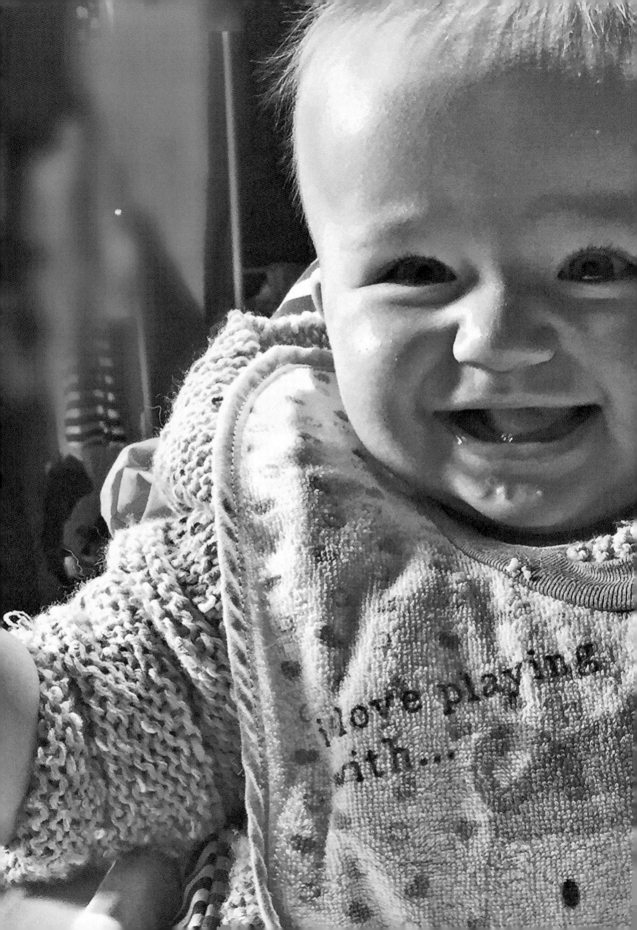

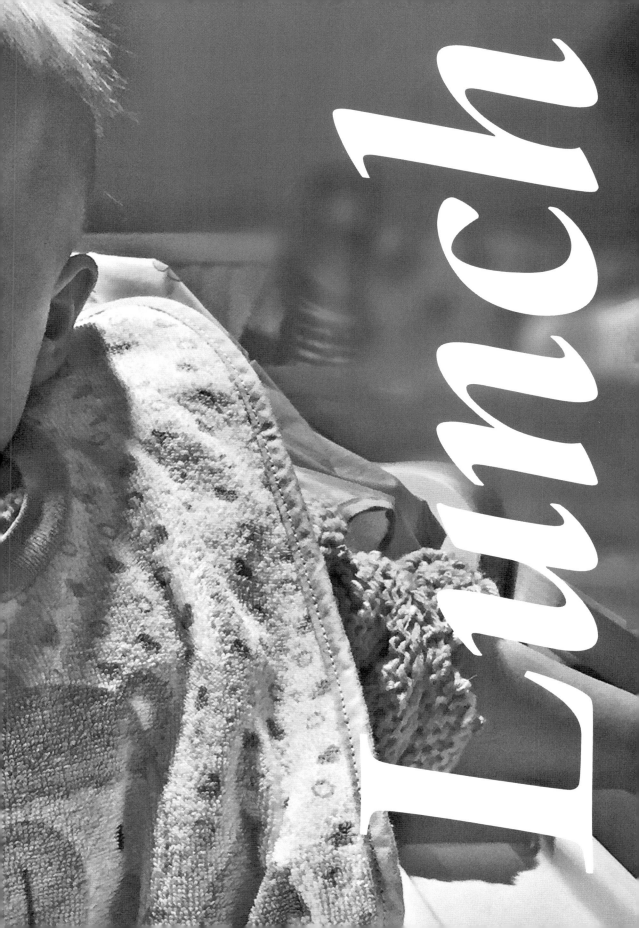

Lunch

Tuna Toastie

This is a really quick lunch idea – the recipe will give you lots of leftover tuna that you can use as topping for sandwiches or jacket potatoes.

- -

Prep Time: 5 mins
Cook Time: 3-5 mins
Yields: 2

- -

Ingredients

4 slices of your preferred bread - I used sourdough
6 tbsp plain yogurt
200g tin of sweetcorn
160g tin of tuna in spring water
Small bowl of grated mild cheddar cheese - or alternative for CMA

- -

Method

- Heat your grill
- Drain tuna and sweetcorn and then mix in a bowl with the yogurt
- Divide tuna mix between 4 slices of bread and top with grated cheese
- Place the tuna bread under the grill for 3-5 minutes until the cheese is melted and golden
- Serve once melted cheese has cooled

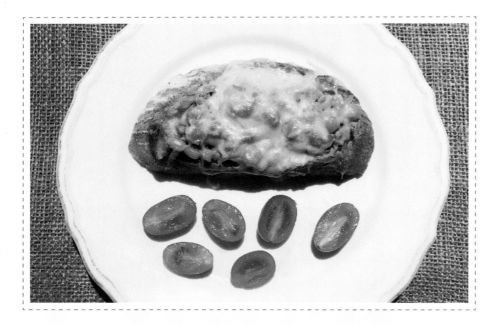

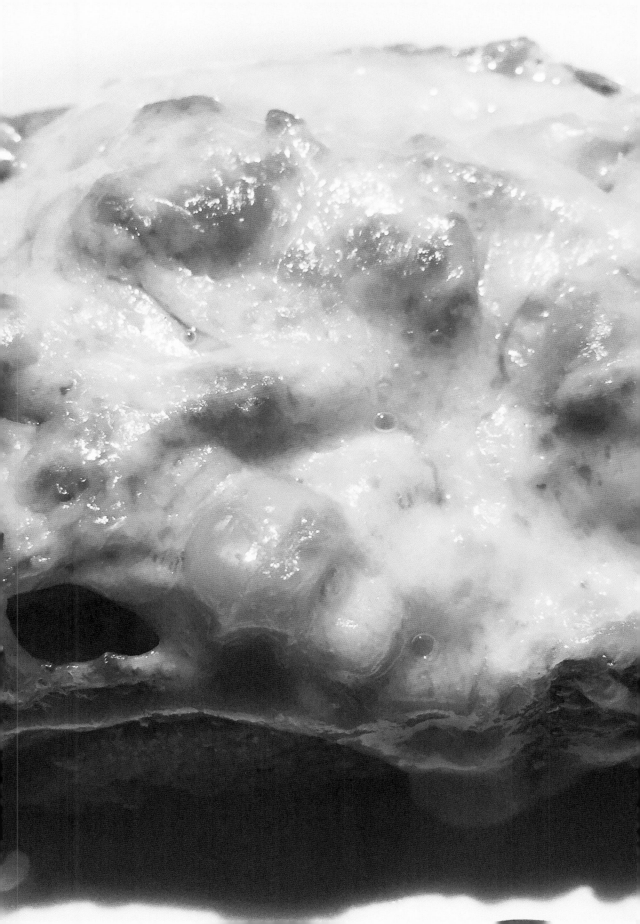

Scotch Pancakes

A quick and easy thick pancake that you can top with a host of delicious toppings.

Prep Time: 10 mins
Cook Time: 4 mins
Yields: 10

Ingredients

1 cup self raising flour
1 egg
150ml milk (soya for cows milk allergy)

Method

- Add the flour to a large bowl - make a well in the middle and break egg into it
- Slowly add the milk - whisking until there are no lumps and you have a smooth thick batter
- Heat oil in a pan and add 2 tablespoons of batter per pancake - fry each pancake for 2 minutes on each side

----

Additional Info

Topping Ideas:
Nutella and fruit
Peanut butter and fruit
Yogurt and fruit puree
Mushed banana
Jam

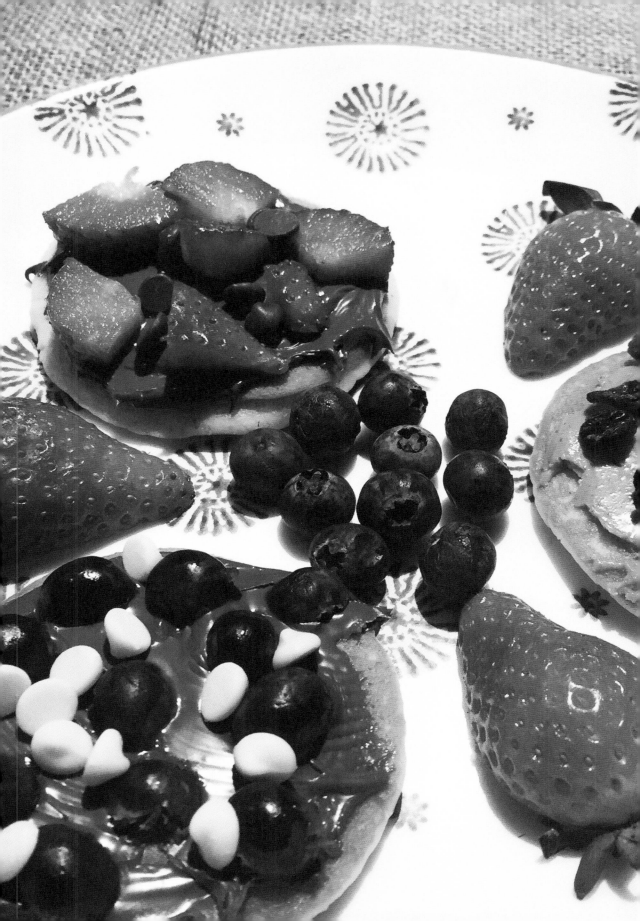

Ham & Cheese Aubergine Bites

These are so delicious Annabelle has to share with me! Since my BLW journey started my love for aubergine has grown immensely – mainly due to my love for my yummy chicken bake (also in this recipe book).

Ingredients

1 aubergine, sliced into 5mm rounds
2 slices of ham cut into 2cm squares
1 1/2 cups of grated mild cheese (or alternative for CMA)
Olive oil

Method

- Heat oven to 180°C
- Place aubergine rounds onto a baking tray
- Drizzle with olive oil and sprinkle with oregano
- Place in the oven and bake for 30-40 minutes until tender.
- Remove aubergine from oven and place ham squares evenly on top of roasted aubergine rounds
- Sprinkle cheese evenly on top of the ham and place under the grill for 3 minutes
- Serve aubergine rounds sliced in half

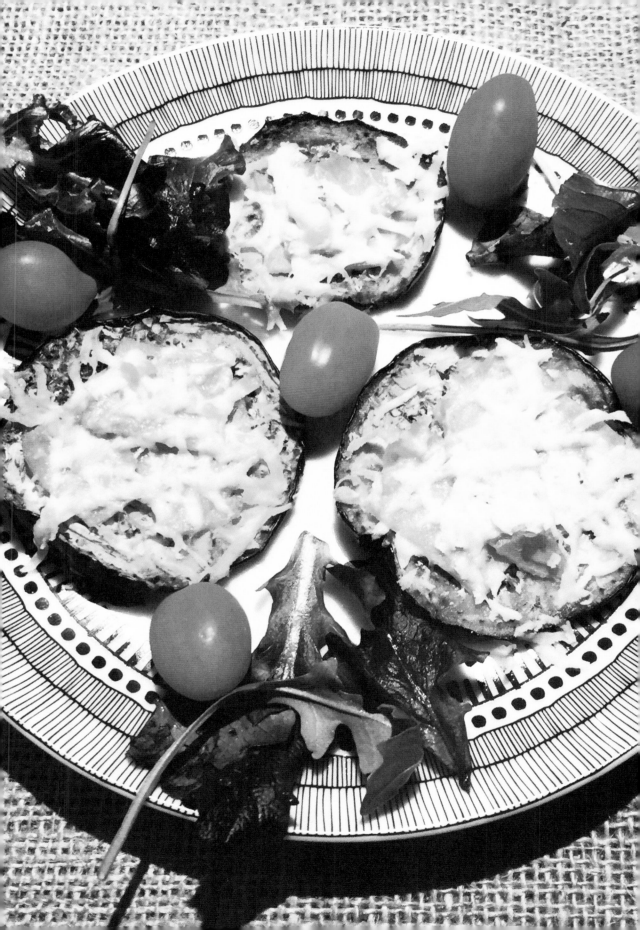

Mini Pizza Bites

A fun idea for lunch or snack time. With so many topping variables your baby can experience a whole host of different flavors and textures.

Ingredients

2 wholemeal or plain tortillas
12 tsp tomato puree
1 1/2 cups of grated cheese (soya for cows milk allergy)
Toppings of your choice

Method

- Heat oven to 190°C
- Simply cut the tortilla into rounds using a scone cutter
- Spread 1 teaspoon of tomato puree on each round - top with grated cheese and toppings of your choice
- Sprinkle with dried oregano and place in the oven on a baking tray for 10-15 minutes until cheese is melted and golden.

Additional Info

Topping ideas: ham and cheese, cheese and sliced mushroom, ham and pineapple, cheese and sweetcorn, beef and diced peppers

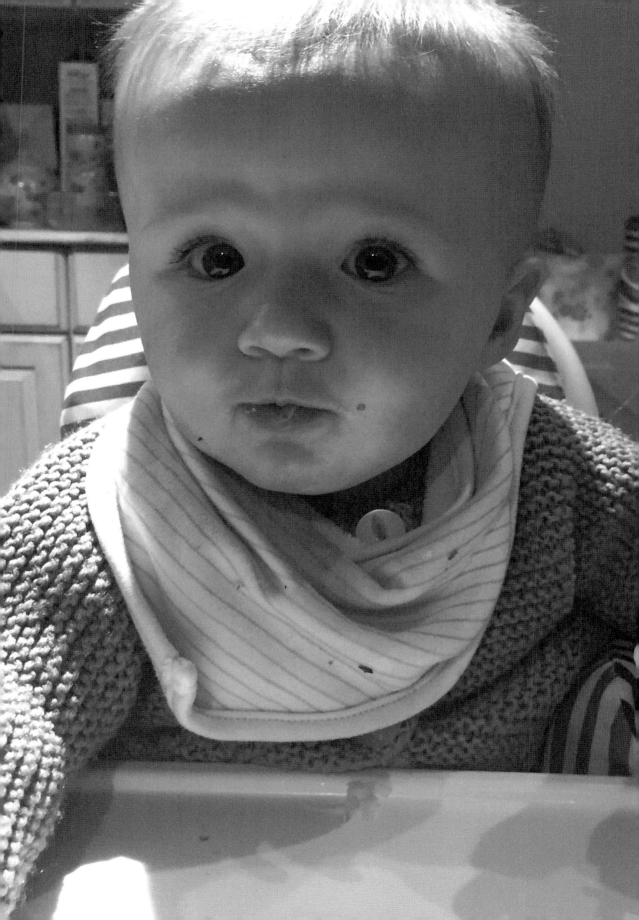

Peanut Butter Wraps

This is our Monday morning snack that also ends up being lunch because Annabelle is simply too tired for a larger lunch after her swimming lesson – I have tried and it was an epic fail. I am usually stressed and in a hurry so she normally has this with some extra fruit (usually strawberries because they are her fav).

- -

Prep Time: 5 mins
Cook Time: 0 mins
Yields: 2

- -

Ingredients

1 plain wholewheat tortilla (or plain if you prefer)

3 tbsp of smooth peanut butter (the Whole Earth brand is fab as it has no added sugar)

1 banana, peeled

- -

Method

- Simple spread the peanut butter all over the tortilla
- Place the peeled banana in the middle of the tortilla and wrap it around
- Slice into 2cm bites.

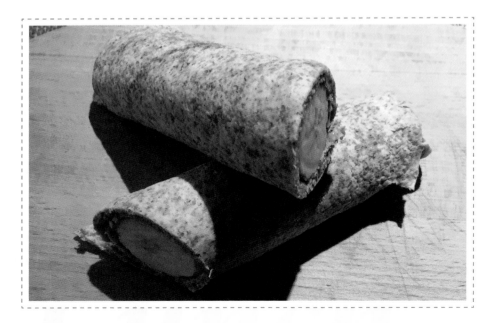

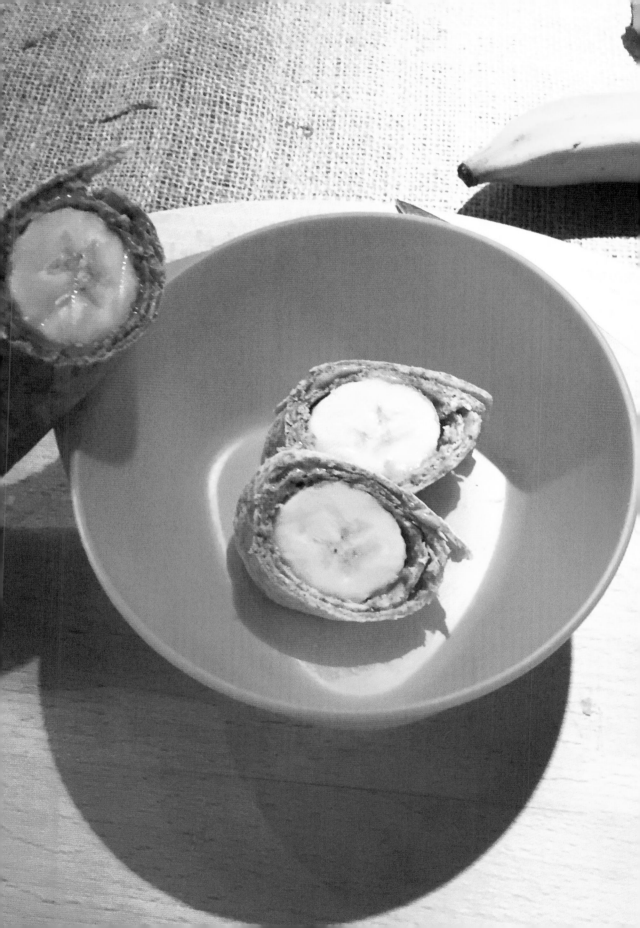

Sourdough Pear Melt

I made this melt one lunchtime when I was at a loose end with not much in the kitchen but some bread and over ripe fruit, it's very simple but so yummy and Annabelle adores it.

- -

Prep Time: 15 mins
Cook Time: 30 mins
Yields: 18

- -

Ingredients

1 slice of sourdough bread
2 slices of pear
3 tbsp of grated cheese
1 heaped tbsp of yogurt
2 pinches of dried mixed herbs

- -

Method

- Simply spoon the yogurt over the sourdough slice - this will help soften it and make it easier for baby to eat
- Place the pear slices on top of the yogurt, sprinkle with cheese and 2 pinches of mixed herbs
- Place the slice under the grill for about 2-3 minutes until the cheese has melted
- Leave to cool before serving

Lunch

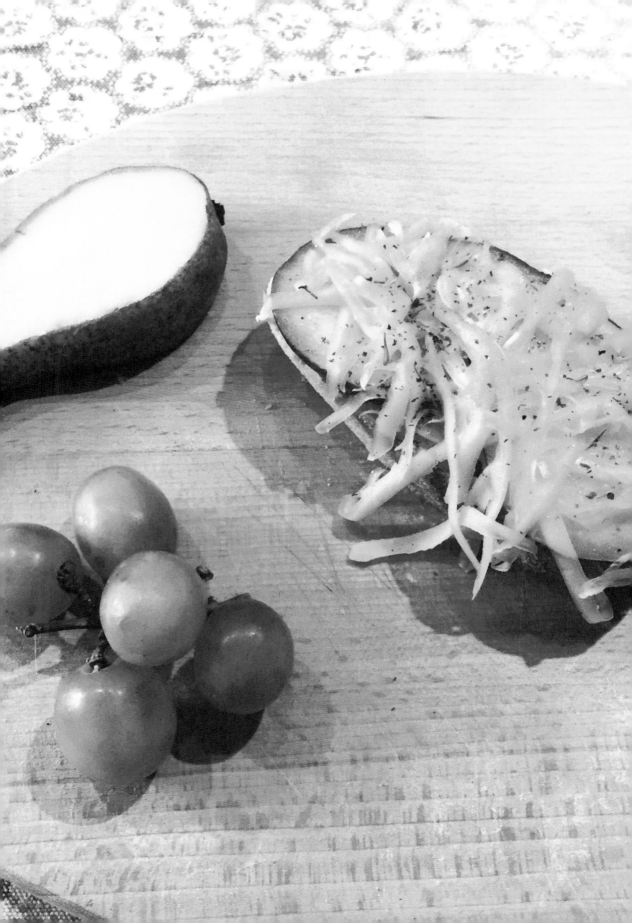

Mini Cranberry & Bacon Rosti's

I am really into Rosti's, the main reason being that both Annabelle and I love them, she loves picking up the smallest of pieces that fall off as she's munching and showing off her very impressive pincer grip!

Prep Time: 15 mins
Cook Time: 12 mins
Yields: 2

Ingredients

1 tbsp plain flour
1 large uncooked baking potato, grated (place in a tea towel and squeeze out excess moisture)
2 rashers of cooked bacon, diced
1 large or 2 small eggs, whisked
2/3 tbsp of cranberry sauce
30g Parmesan cheese (or soya cheese for cows milk allergy)

Method

- Mix all of the ingredients in a large bowl
- Add 3 tablespoons (use image as guide) to a hot frying pan and fry on rosti on each side for 5 minutes (you should be able to fit 3 per pan)
- Add rosti's to heated plate and continue until you have used all mix... enjoy!

Additional Info

These can be stored in the fridge for up to 3 days and heated up in the oven or microwave

Lunch

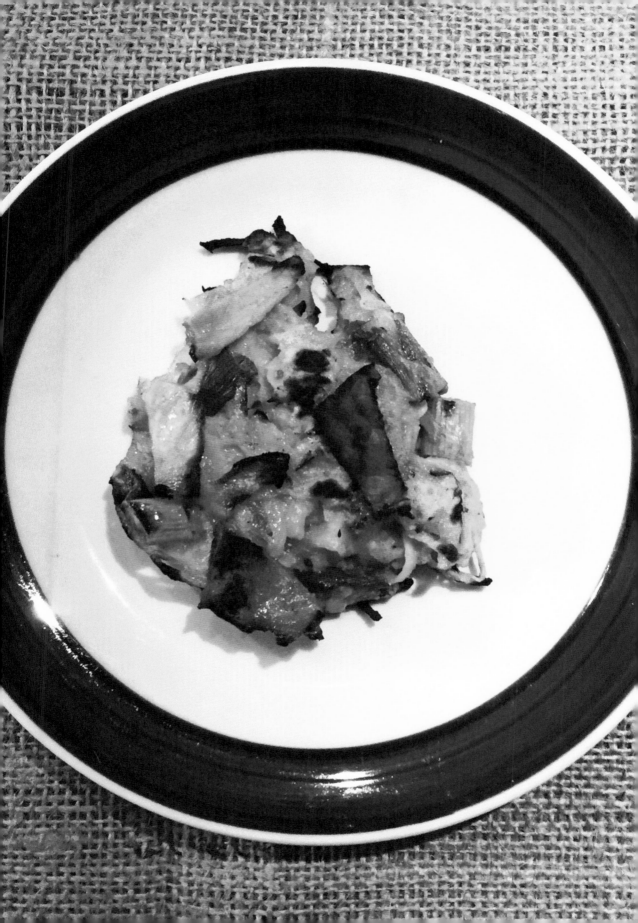

Peanut Butter Soldiers

Prep Time: 5 mins
Cook Time: 0 mins
Yields: 1

Ingredients

1 slice wholemeal bread
1 tomato
Peanut butter
Butter (optional)

Method

- Simply spread peanut butter onto wholemeal bread and cut into soldiers
- Serve with tomato wedges

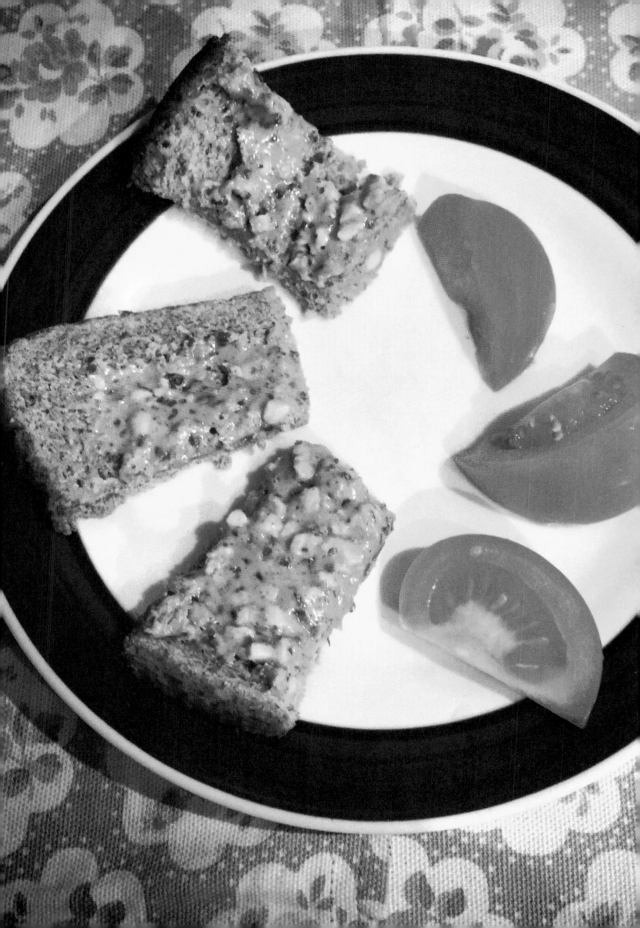

Cranberry, Bacon & Cheese Rolls

This is a very naughty but very delicious lunch, your baby will simply adore these but try not to offer them too often as they are quite salty. Bacon can be substituted for cooked chicken, turkey or ham. Try not to worry about the fat content, unlike us adults babies need a high fat diet.

Prep Time: 10 mins
Cook Time: 40 mins
Yields: 11

Ingredients

4 rashers of bacon
1 cup of grated mild cheese
1/2 cup cranberry sauce
1 pre-rolled sheet of puff pastry

Method

- Grill bacon until cooked through, remove and set aside
- Roll out puff pastry and spread cranberry sauce evenly across the whole width of the pastry
- Once bacon has cooled, finely chop into 2 cm approx. chunks and scatter over the cranberry sauce - top with grated cheese
- Roll up the pastry sheet lengthways and then cut into rolls every 2.5 cm's.
- Place rolls onto a lined baking tray and bake for 15 -25 mins checking often. Pastry should be golden and cheese melting from the sides slightly.
- Serve to baby once cooled

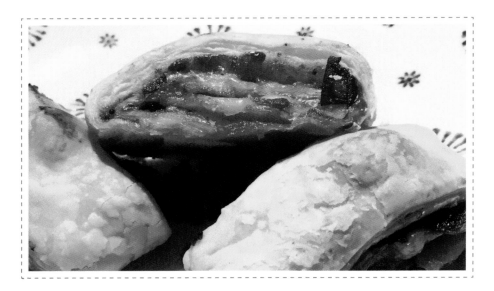

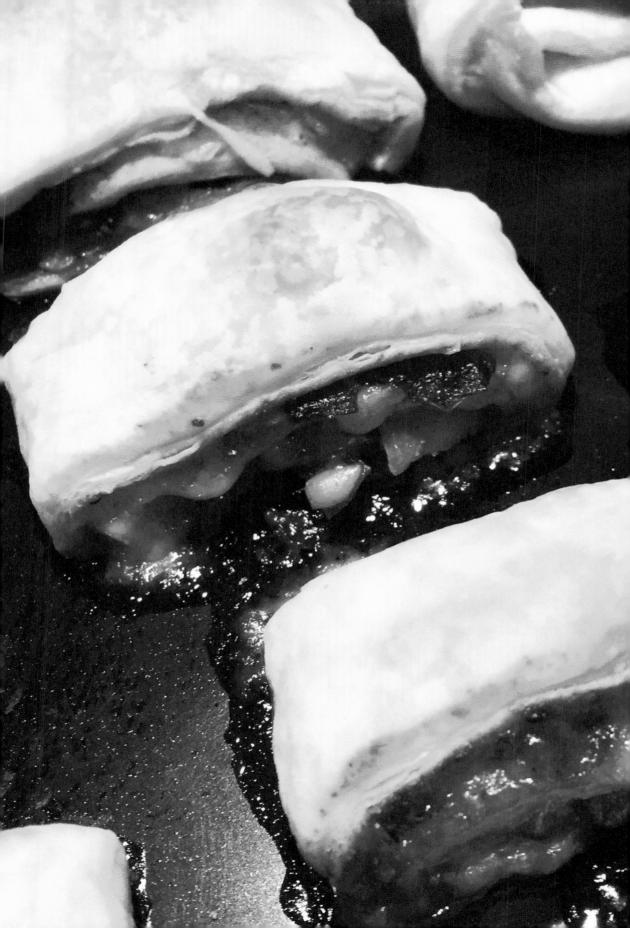

More Lunch Ideas

Tuna mixed with plain full fat or soya yogurt on toast or bread

Pate on toast or bread

Scrambled egg made with full fat butter on toast

Mushed Avocado on toast

Chopped or mushed banana on toast

Toast fingers

Cheese on toast (with cranberry sauce optional)

Simple beef, chicken or turkey sandwich

Tuna sandwich

Egg sandwich

Ham and cheese toasty

Cranberry and turkey sandwiches

Scrambled egg on toast

Pitta pizza

Pork sandwiches with apple sauce

Fried egg on toast

Hard boiled egg and toast soldiers

Fruit salad with cheese slices

Crumpet with butter and/or jam

Toast with ricotta and choice or fruit slices as topping

Toast with Nutella and mushed or sliced banana

A selection of fruit slices, cheese slices and meat slices

Lunch

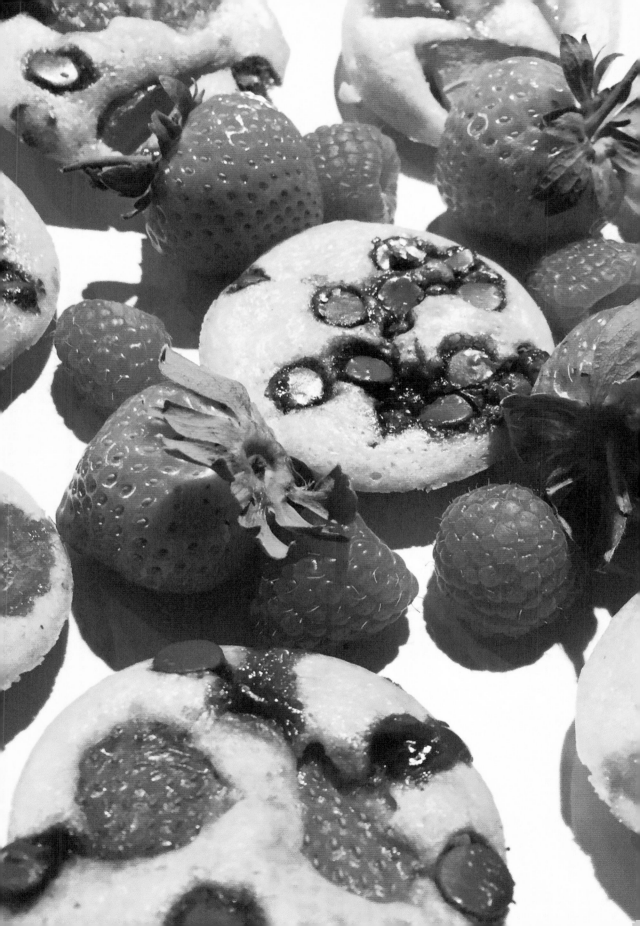

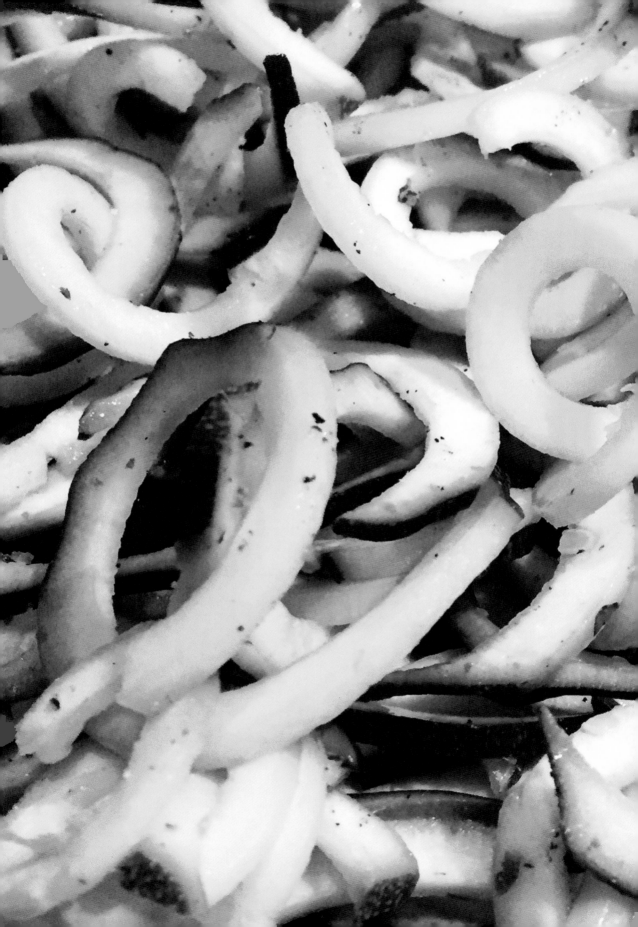

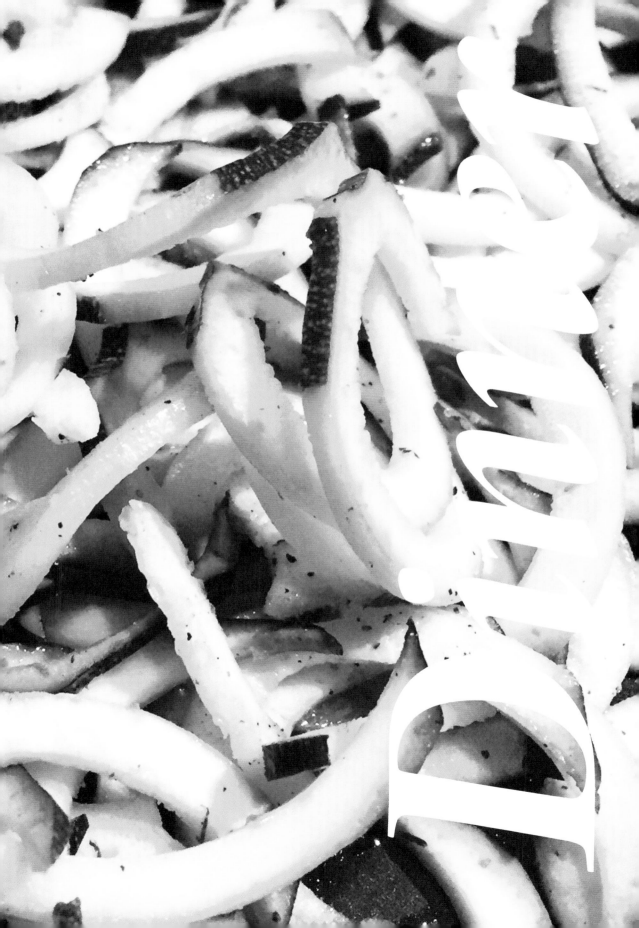

Courgetti Bolognese
(can be made with spaghetti)

Prep Time: 20 mins
Cook Time: 50 mins
Yields: 4

Ingredients

2 courgettes, spirilizer used the 'noodle' setting OR 300g spaghetti pasta
400g/14oz beef mince
1 onion, finely diced
2 garlic cloves, chopped OR 2 tbsp minced garlic
100g/3½oz carrot, cut into small 0.5mm cubes
2 x 400g tin chopped tomatoes
400ml/14fl oz low salt beef stock
2 tbsp Worcestershire sauce
Black pepper to season

Method

- Place carrots into a microwave safe bowl, cover with water and microwave for 5 minutes. Drain and set aside
- Fry mince until browned, drain excess fat and set aside
- In the same frying pan fry the onion for 6 minutes, then add garlic and carrots and cook for a further 2 minutes
- Return the mince to the pan and add tomatoes, stock, Worcestershire sauce and a good grind of black pepper - allow to simmer for 45 minutes
- Once mince has simmered for 45 minutes, turn heat off and simply fry courgetti over a medium heat for 5 minutes
- Serve to baby once cooled

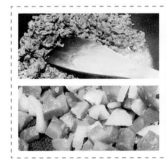
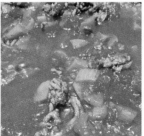
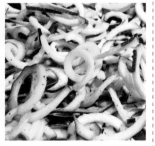

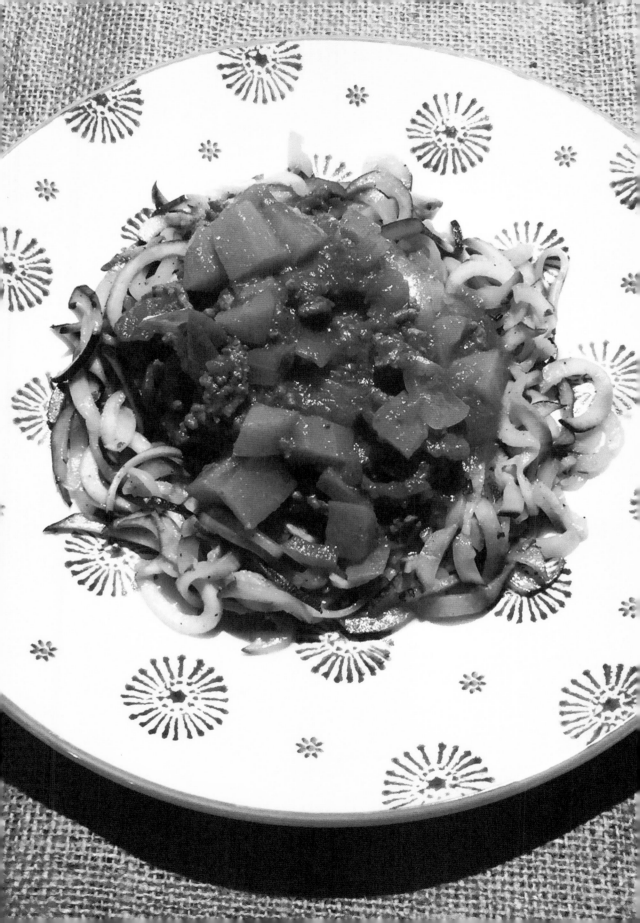

Bubble and Squeak Bake

Prep Time: 20 mins
Cook Time: 25 mins
Yields: 4

Ingredients

2 potatoes, peeled and cut into 8 (think roast potato size or a bit smaller)
1 whole cabbage - heads broken from stalk
2 carrots, peeled and diced
1 1/2 cup of grated mild cheese (or alternative for CMA)
3 large knobs of unsalted butter
1 tsp black pepper
2 eggs, whisked

Method

- Preheat oven to 180 °C
- Place all chopped ingredients into a large saucepan of boiling water, let veg boil for 25 minutes
- Add pepper, butter and mash veg, stir through the cheese and then allow mix to cool completely
- Once cool stir through the whisked eggs and transfer to a large baking dish
- Sprinkle with cheese and bake for 30 minutes until golden
- Serve to baby once cooled

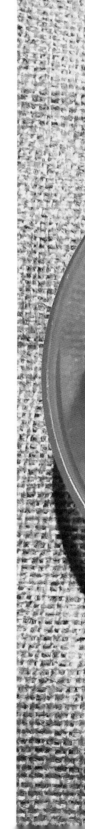

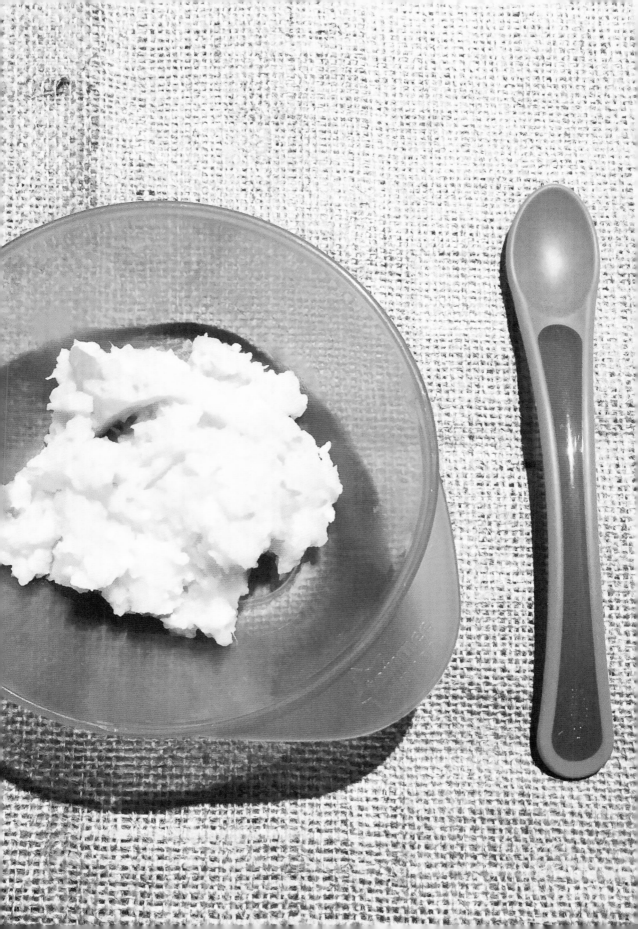

Sweet Meat Loaf

Prep Time: 15 mins
Cook Time: 2 hours
Yields: 6

Ingredients

2 lbs ground beef
1/2 tsp garlic powder
1 onion, finely diced
1 egg
1/2 tsp black pepper
1/4 cup brown sugar
1 cup Ritz crackers, ground to fine crumbs in a food processor
1 cup full fat milk
1/4 cup apricot jam
1 1/4 cup reduced salt tomato ketchup
1 tbsp Worcestershire sauce

Method

- Heat oven to 180°C and line a 9"x5" loaf tray
- In a large bowl mix beef, crackers, egg, milk, 1/2 cup ketchup, onion, pepper and garlic powder
- Pour mix into a lined loaf tin and bake for 1 hour
- Meanwhile combine 3/4 ketchup, brown sugar, apricot jam and worcestershire sauce -
- After the meatloaf has been baking for 1 hour, pour the above mix onto the meat loaf and spread evenly. Return loaf to the oven and bake for a further 30 minutes
- Serve to baby once cooled

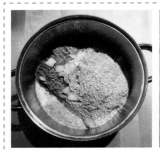 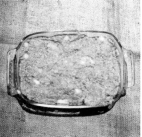 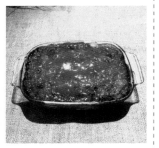

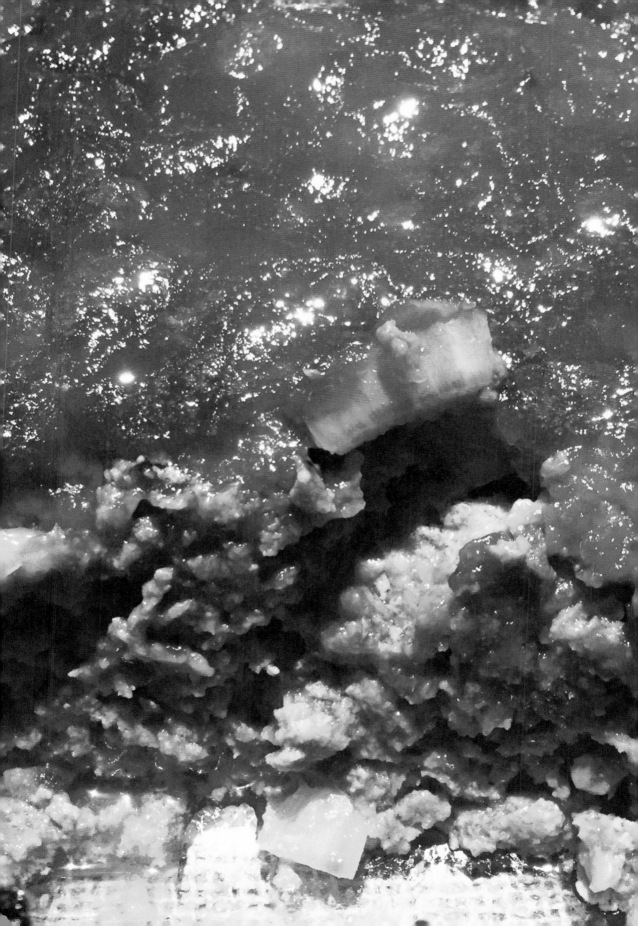

Chicken Parmigiana with Smoky Carrot Fries

This is a very easy cheat meal that Annabelle and I love, we enjoy it when daddy is away as he can't stand parmesan cheese. I used 'fry light' to keep calories as low as possible for me. You could add some potatoes cooked the same way as the carrot fries if you would like to increase the carbs for bub.

- -

Prep Time: 5 mins
Cook Time: 30 mins
Yields: 4

- -

Ingredients

8 carrots, chopped into french fries
4 shop brought breaded chicken steaks
4 tbsp tomato puree
1/2 cup parmesan cheese (or soya for cows milk allergy)
2 tbsp of paprika

- -

Method

- Heat oven to 180°C
- Add carrot fries to baking tray (you may need 2) and drizzle with olive oil/ sprinkle with paprika
- Place in the oven and set timer for 20 minutes
- Once the timer has buzzed keep the carrots cooking in the oven and start frying your chicken steaks for 4 minutes on each side
- Once chicken steaks are warmed through spread 1 tbsp of tomato puree on one side of each steak and top with parmesan cheese
- Place chicken steaks under the grill for 3-5 minutes until parmesan is starting to melt
- Your carrots should now be nicely cooked through and slightly crispy.
- Serve chicken and carrot fries for baby slightly cooled.

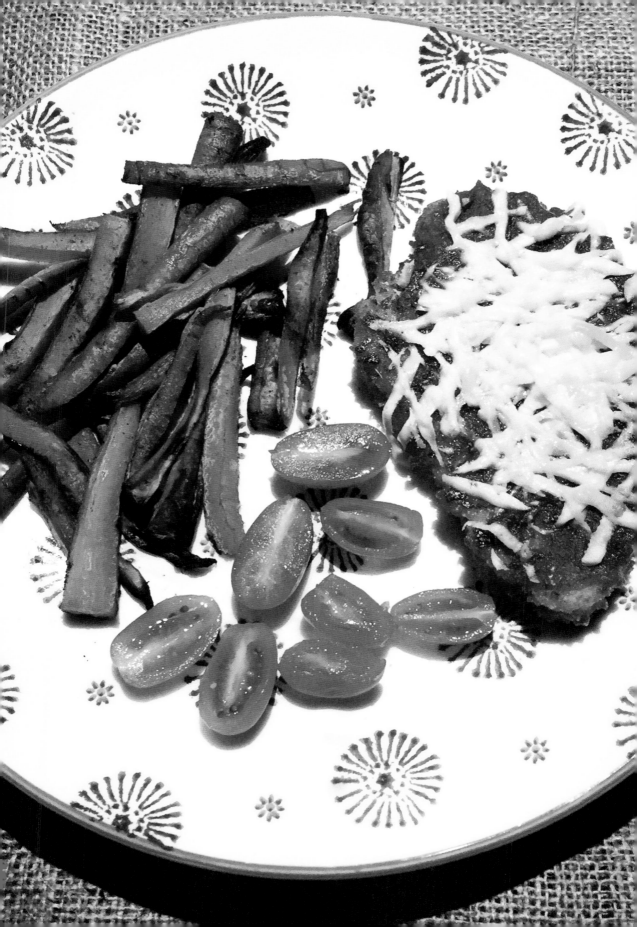

Turkey Pasta Bake

This recipe is adapted from a very old Weight Watchers book that my mother in law gave to me after Annabelle was born, it was the first meal we ate when we got home from the birthing center and although it was a challenge to eat as Annabelle and her reflux meant she couldn't be put down I really enjoyed it.

- -

Prep Time: 20 mins
Cook Time: 30 mins
Yields: 4

- -

Ingredients

225 g turkey mince, raw
1 small onion, chopped
2 cloves garlic, crushed
1 medium red pepper, de-seeded and chopped
400 g chopped tinned tomatoes
100ml low salt chicken stock
85g penne pasta, dry
1 teaspoons (level) oregano, dried
1/4 teaspoon black pepper
25g to sprinkle on top when serving

- -

Method

- Heat oven to 180°C
- Heat oil in a frying pan until hot and then fry the minced turkey, stirring well for approx. 8 minutes, or until cooked and crumbly
- Add the onion, garlic, pepper and oil. Mix well, cover and cook for 5 minutes, until the vegetables have softened.
- Stir in the tomatoes, stock or water, pasta shapes, herbs and seasoning. Bring to the boil and simmer for 2 minutes.
- Spoon the mixture into a small casserole dish. Cover and bake for 30 minutes.
- Uncover and serve once cooled, sprinkled with the grated cheese.

- -

Additional Info

This meal is especially delicious with lamb or beef mince which also has the added benefit of being iron rich.

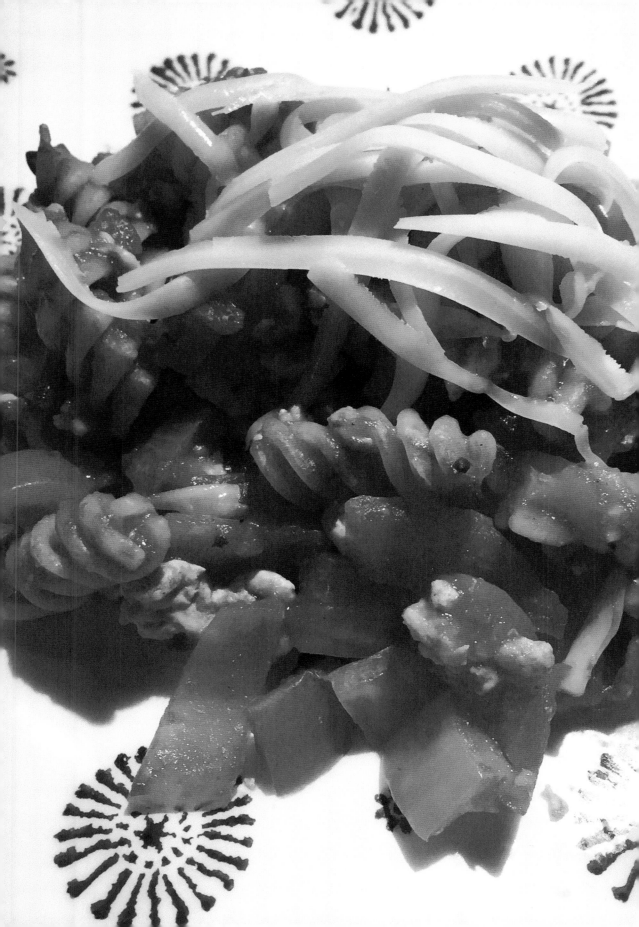

Annabelle's Chicken Korma

I make this chicken korma in my slow cooker but to make it in a conventional oven I would suggest using a large casserole dish and cooking for 40mins at 200 degrees. However this is only using my best judgement so please ensure you check chicken is cooked thoroughly before serving.

Prep Time: 25 mins
Cook Time: 8 hours
Yields: 4

Ingredients

4 chicken breasts diced
2 onions, finely chopped
1 green chilli, deseeded and finely chopped
2 tbsp of ginger paste
6 tbsp of korma curry paste
250ml of tinned coconut cream
300ml low salt chicken stock
3 heaped tbsp ground almonds
handful of fresh coriander, roughly chopped

Method

- Heat oil in a pan and cook chicken in batches until golden, place into slow cooker
- Now simply add all other ingredients to the slow cooker, place the lid on top and cook for 8 hours on LOW

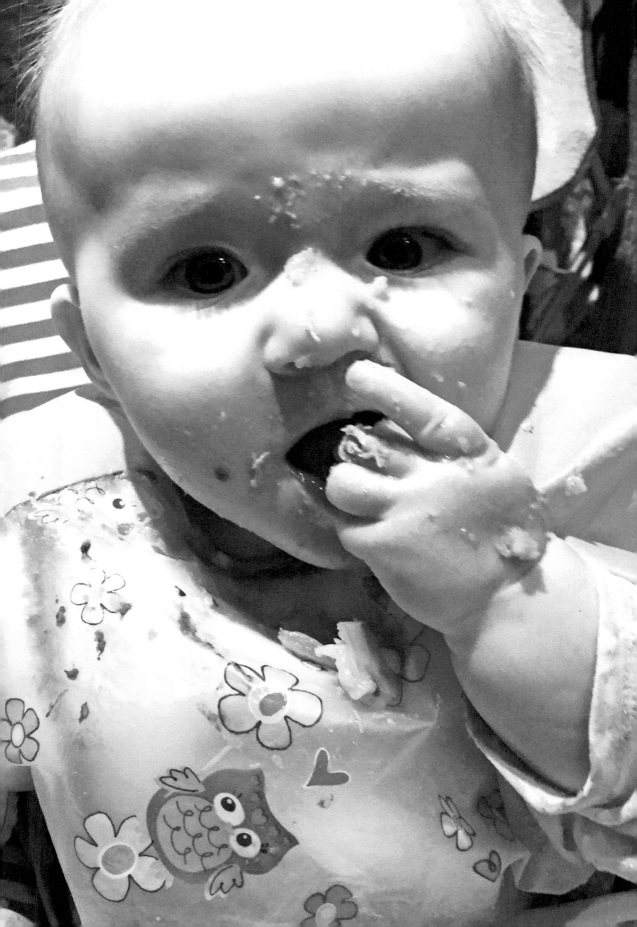

Super Mild Chilli Con Carne

Once I had tried Annabelle on chicken korma (and her loving it!) I became a lot more confident giving her more flavorsome foods that I already enjoy with hubby. That's what I really love most about baby led weaning is that Annabelle can eat the same as us for the most part – it saves so much time!

Prep Time: 25 mins
Cook Time: 40 mins
Yields: 4

Ingredients

500g lean beef mince
1 onion, diced
1 small sweet potato, diced
1 small green pepper, diced
4 celery stalks, sliced
4-5 mushrooms, diced
1 large carrot, diced
1 x 400g tins red kidney beans, drained
1 x 400g tin chopped tomatoes
1 cup vegetable stock
1 cup beef stock
1 tsp sugar
1 cup water
1 tsp mild chilli powder
1 tsp paprika

Method

- In a large sauce pan fry the onion and pepper until softened. Once soft add the beef and cook until browned
- Now simply add all other ingredients and cook covered over a medium heat for 30 minutes
- Serve with rice, pasta or in tortilla wraps.

Dinner

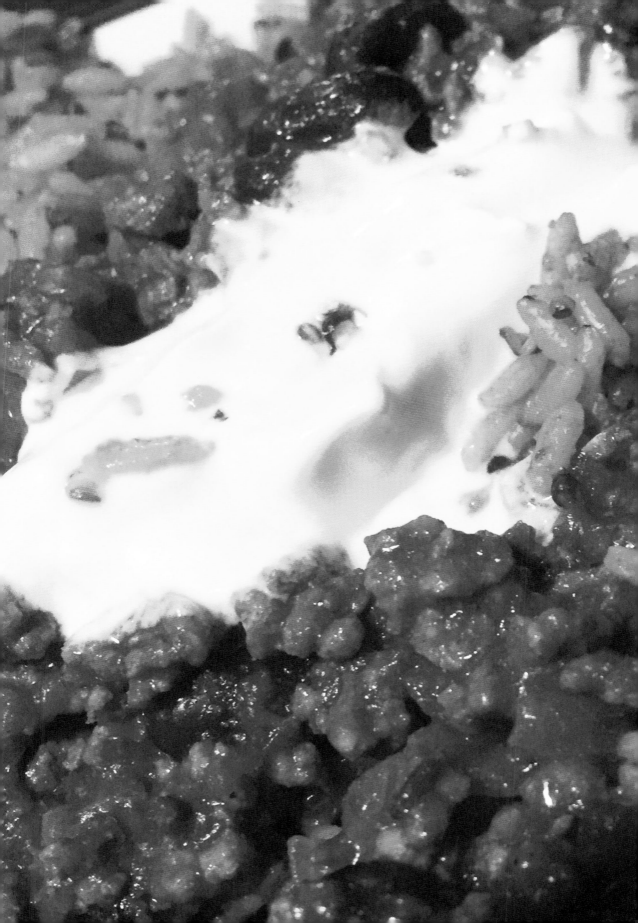

Simple Shepherds Pie

Hearty, wholesome, deliciousness is how I can best describe this shepherds pie – Annabelle adores anything with mince so this meal is a sure fire winner!

The cheese in this recipe is optional but it makes it simply irresistible and I personally can not resist!

- -

Prep Time: 20 mins
Cook Time: 1 hour
Yields: 4

- -

Ingredients

1 large onion chopped
8 mushrooms sliced
2-3 medium carrots, diced into very small chunks
500g pack lamb mince
2 tbsp tomato purée
1 tbsp worcestershire sauce
500ml low salt beef stock
900g potato, cut into chunks
85g butter
3 tbsp milk
2 cups of grated mild cheese

- -

Method

- Heat oil in a large pan and add onions and carrots - fry for 5 minutes until soft.
- Once soft add the mushrooms and crumble in the lamb mince - cook until browned
- Once the mince has browned pour in the stock, Worcestershire sauce and tomato purée and simmer for 30 minutes
- Heat oven to 180 and start boiling potatoes ready to make the mash. Boil potatoes for 10-15 mins until tender. Drain, then mash with the butter and milk (soya for CMA).
- Place mince in overproof dish and top with mashed potato. Top with a generous grating of mild cheese and bake for 30 minutes.

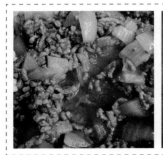 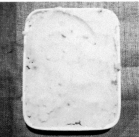 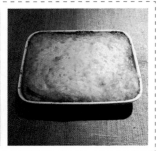

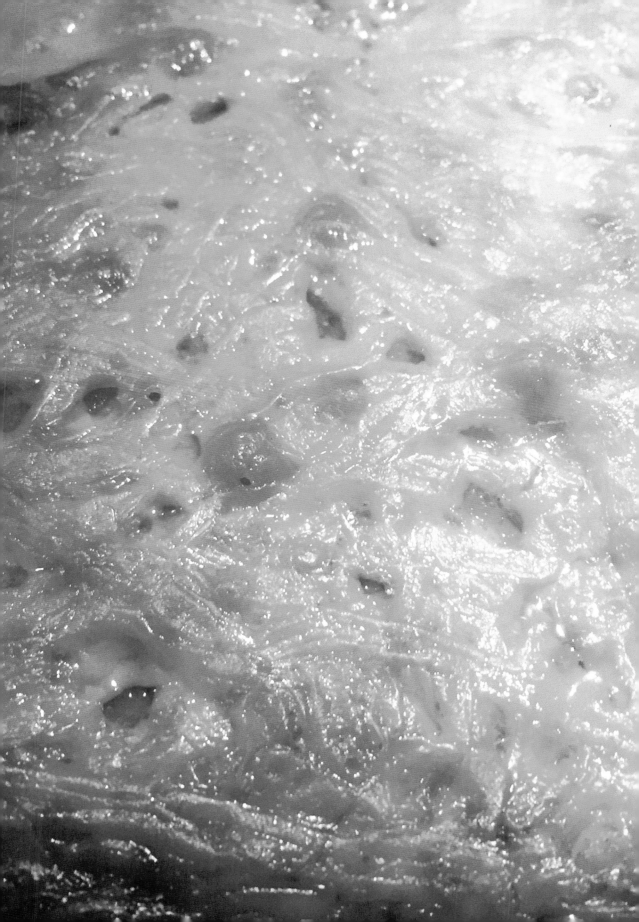

Veggie Pizza

This delicious veggie tortilla pizza is a life saver when you need a healthy meal in record time.

- -

Prep Time: 15 mins
Cook Time: 15 mins
Yields: 2

- -

Ingredients

2 wholemeal flour tortillas
One handful of mushrooms, sliced
4 cooked broccoli heads, roughly chopped
4 cooked cauliflower heads, roughly chopped
10 tbsp of passata, leftovers can be used to make a simple pasta sauce*
1/2 white onion, diced
1 tbsp oregano
Grated cheese (soya variety for cows milk allergy)
4 slices of cooked beef cut into strips

- -

Method

- Heat oven to 180°C
- Add diced onion to a frying pan and cook until soft (about 5 minutes), add mushrooms and fry for a further 2 minutes
- Turn off the heat and add the cooked beef, cauliflower, broccoli and oregano - stir to combine
- Spoon passata over both tortillas, spreading evenly like pizza sauce*
- Evenly spoon half of the onion mix onto each tortilla
- Top with a generous sprinkling of grated cheese and place in preheated oven for 10-15 minutes.

- -

Additional Info

* LEFTOVER PASSATA 1.Simply pour passata into a jug and mix in 3 heaped tbsp of tomato puree - mix well 2. Next stir in 1 TSP of Oregano and half a teaspoon of brown sugar and you have a easy peasy pasta sauce 3. Simple stir into cooked pasta and serve! (Leftovers can be frozen in ice cube trays)

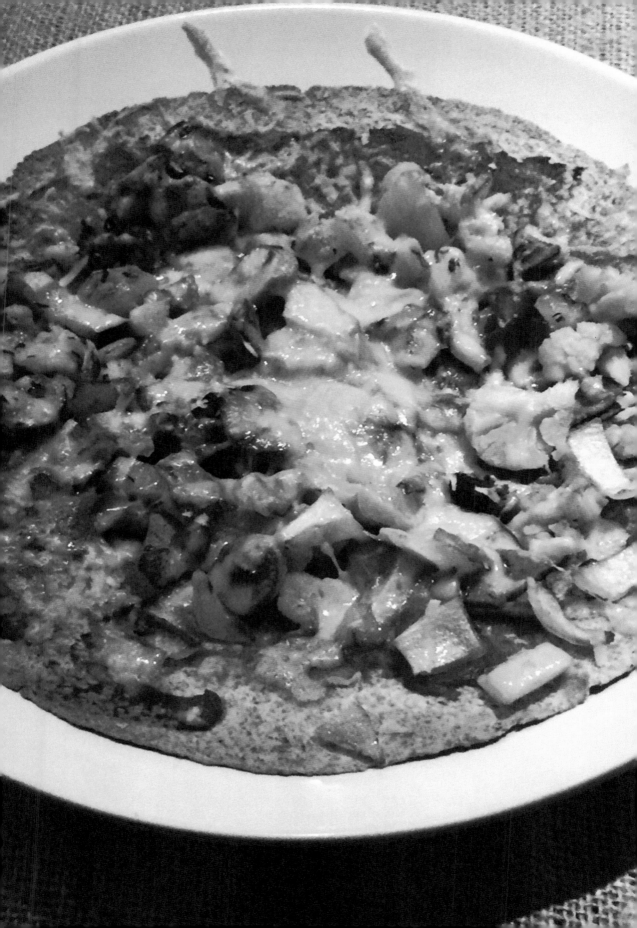

Chicken Rosti

This recipe is brilliant because your more than likely to have the ingredients on hand! And if you don't have spring onion you can swap them for half an onion and you can use pretty much use meat you like. This dish will serve 1 adult and 1 baby/child

- -

Prep Time: 15 mins
Cook Time: 12 mins
Yields: 2

- -

Ingredients

1 tbsp plain flour
1 large uncooked baking potato, grated (place in a tea towel and squeeze out excess moisture)
5 spring onions, finely sliced
1 large or 2 small eggs, whisked
1 cooked chicken breast, diced
30g Parmesan cheese (or soya cheese for cows milk allergy)
50g frozen peas or sweetcorn (I used peas) but sweetcorn might be better for fussy eaters
Black pepper to season
Olive oil for frying

- -

Method

- Mix all ingredients in a large bowl
- Add the potato mix to a frying pan pushing down to form a large patty - fry on a medium heat for 5 minutes
- Using a plate flip patty and fry for another 5 minutes

Dinner

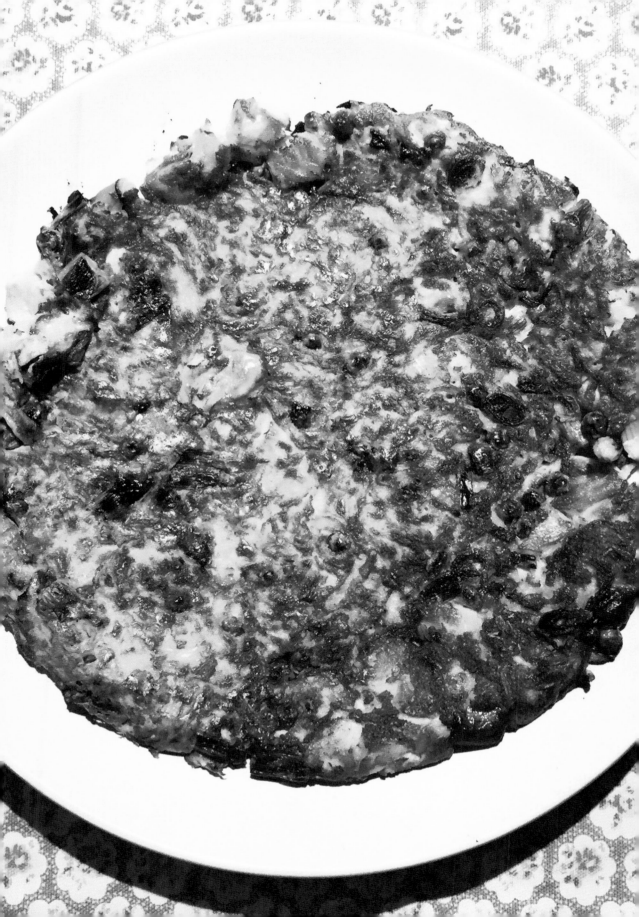

Chicken Bake

Prep Time: 20 mins
Cook Time: 60 mins
Yields: 4

Ingredients

1 aubergine, thinly sliced
4 chicken breasts, cut into slices
1 courgette, cut into chunks
2 tomatoes, cut into wedges
1/2 punnet cherry tomatoes, cut in half lengthways
6 button mushrooms, sliced
1 cup black olives, cut in half
1/8 cup dried oregano
1/8 cup dried mixed herbs
600ml passata
3 tablespoons balsamic vinegar
3 tablespoons brown sugar
1 tbsp garlic powder
2 garlic cloves crushed

Method

- Heat oven to 180°C
- Add aubergine and courgette to the bottom of an ovenproof dish
- Top with chicken , garlic powder, tomatoes, olives, oregano, mixed herbs and mushrooms
- In a bowl mix passata, vinegar and sugar and then pour on top of chicken and vegetables.
- Bake for 1 hour

Additional Info

Serve with couscous or brown rice.

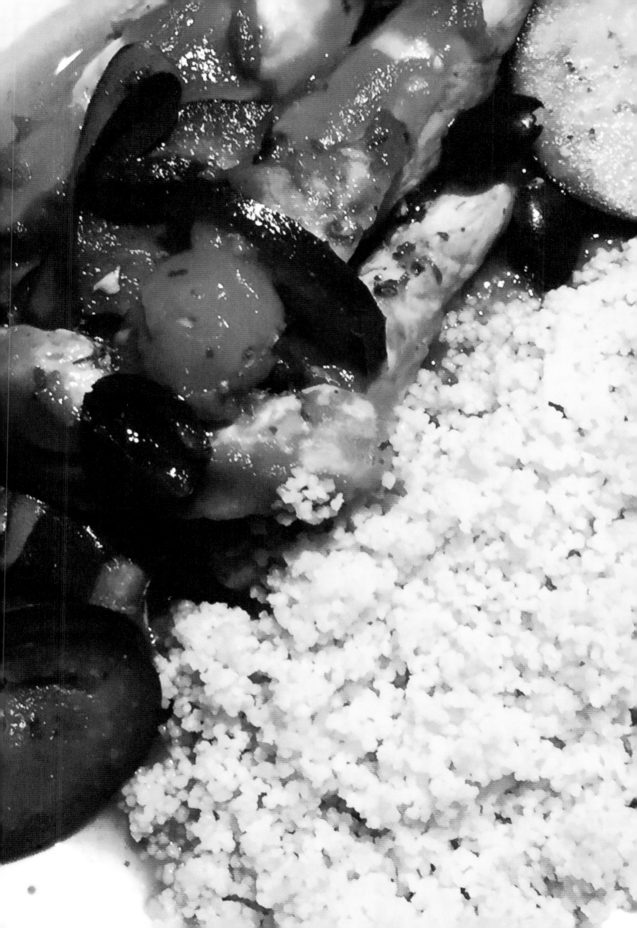

Timesaving Tortilla Pizza

This deliciously simple meal is inspired by the wonderful Annabel Karmel. It's wonderful those evening your simply too frazzled to cook a complex meal.

- -

Prep Time: 15 mins
Cook Time: 15 mins
Yields: 2

- -

Ingredients

2 wholemeal flour tortillas
One handful of mushrooms, sliced
One handful of cherry tomatoes, cut in half lengthways
2 Large tomatoes, Sliced
10 tbsp of passata, leftovers can be used to make a simple pasta sauce*
Grated cheese (soya variety for cows milk allergy)
1 cooked chicken breast, cut into slices

- -

Method

- Heat oven to 190°C/fan 170°C/gas 5
- Simply spoon passata over both tortillas, spreading evenly like pizza sauce
- Scatter chicken, mushrooms and tomatoes on top of passata
- Top with a generous sprinkling of grated cheese and place in preheated oven for 10-15 minutes.

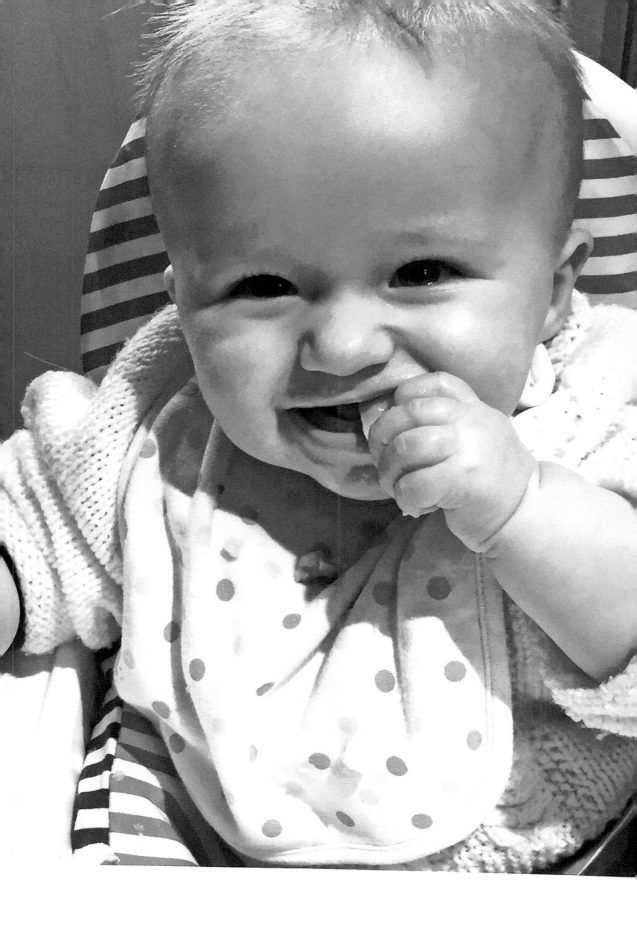

Pear, Pea & Brussels Sprout Pasta

This is such an easy dish to whip up and leftovers can be batched up and frozen for a later date. It's ideal for fussy eaters as the pear gives the dish a super sweet flavor.

Prep Time: 15 mins
Cook Time: 20 mins
Yields: 4

Ingredients

350g dried fussili pasta
3 pears, peeled and quartered - pips removed
2 cups of frozen peas
A small handful of brussels sprouts (about 7)
Parmesan cheese to serve (or soya for cows milk allergy) - optional

Method

- Start by cooking the dried pasta in boiling water as per packet instructions - usually 12 mins
- In the meantime steam peas, pears and brussels sprouts. After 4 mins transfer peas and pear to food processor and continue to steam brussels sprouts
- Once buzzer goes off for the pasta, remove both pasta and brussels sprouts from the heat, drain pasta and set aside
- Add brussels sprouts to food processor along with the pear and peas and blitz to create a lumpy sauce
- Simply stir the sauce and through the pasta and serve plain or with cheese

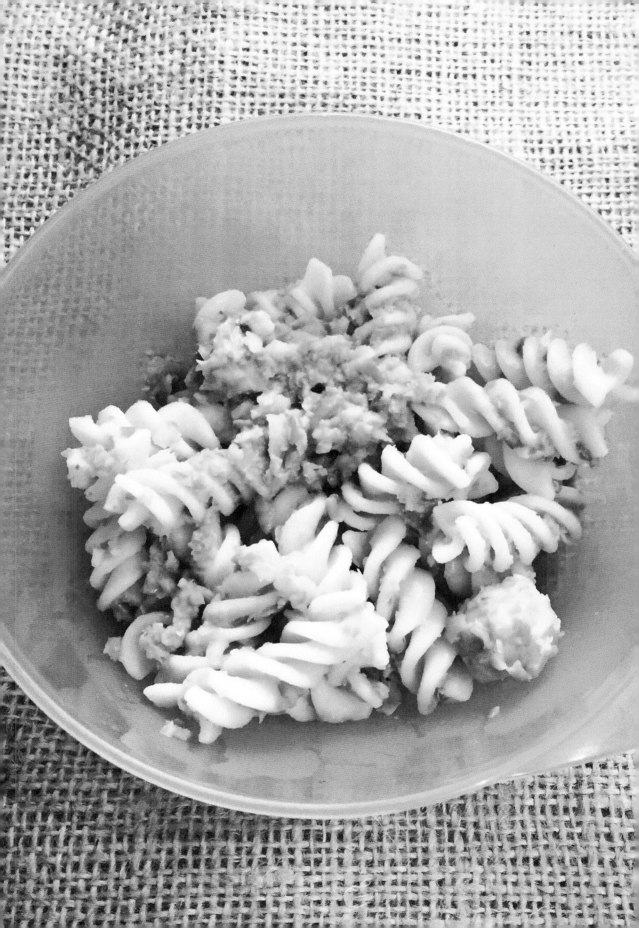

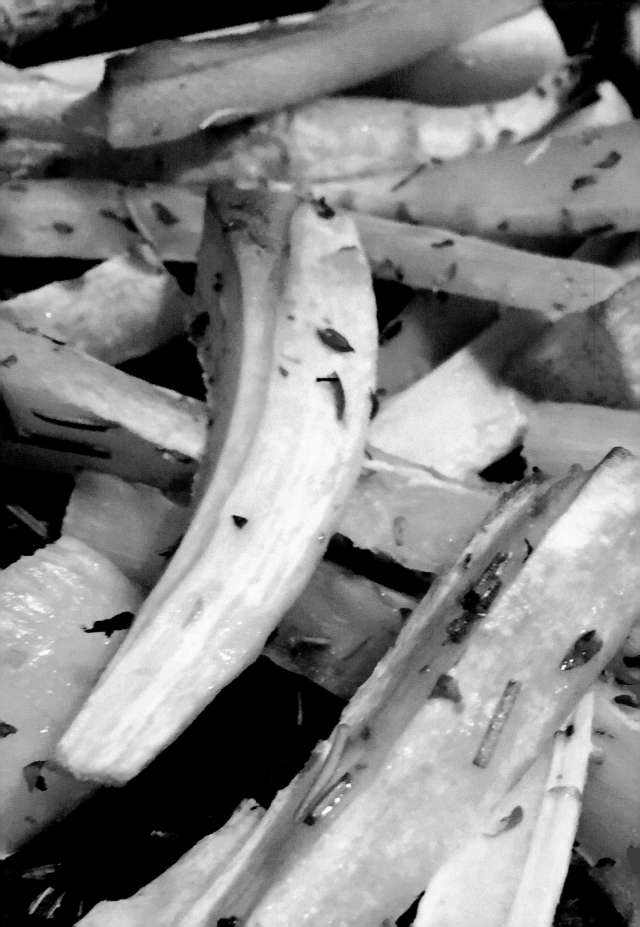

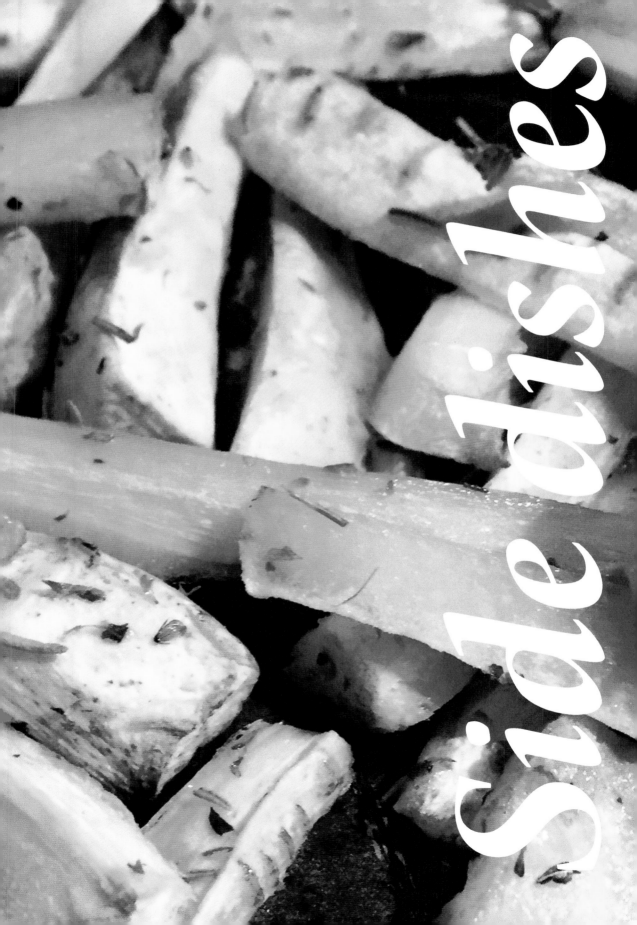

Side dishes

Sweet Potato Noodles

A healthy alternative to spaghetti and it's so sweet and delicious!

- -

Prep Time: 15 mins
Cook Time: 10 mins
Yields: 2

- -

Ingredients

1 sweet potato
Olive oil for frying

- -

Method

- ■ Spiralize your sweet potato using your the spiralizer's 'spiralize' grater
- ■ Heat olive oil in a pan and fry noodles for for 7-10 minutes

- -

Additional Info

Ideal served with slices of meat

Side dishes

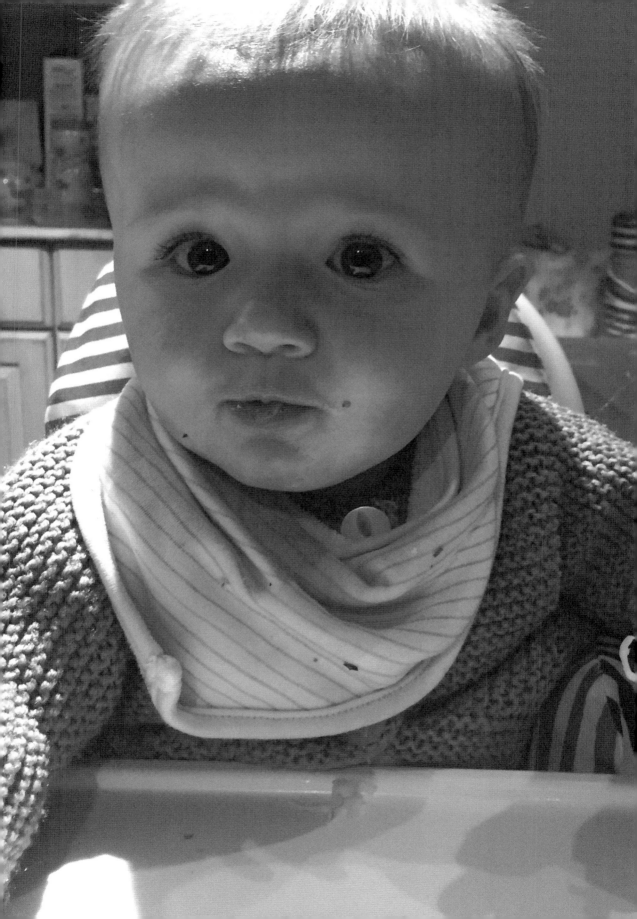

Cauliflower Mash

This makes a lovely change to traditional mashed potato. Perfect served on a pre-loaded spoon.

Prep Time: 15 mins
Cook Time: 30 mins
Yields: 18

Ingredients

2 cauliflowers, chopped from stalk
2 garlic cloves

Method

- Steam garlic and cauliflowers for 5-10 minutes until cauliflower is tender
- Blend or mash cauliflower and garlic until smooth

Side dishes

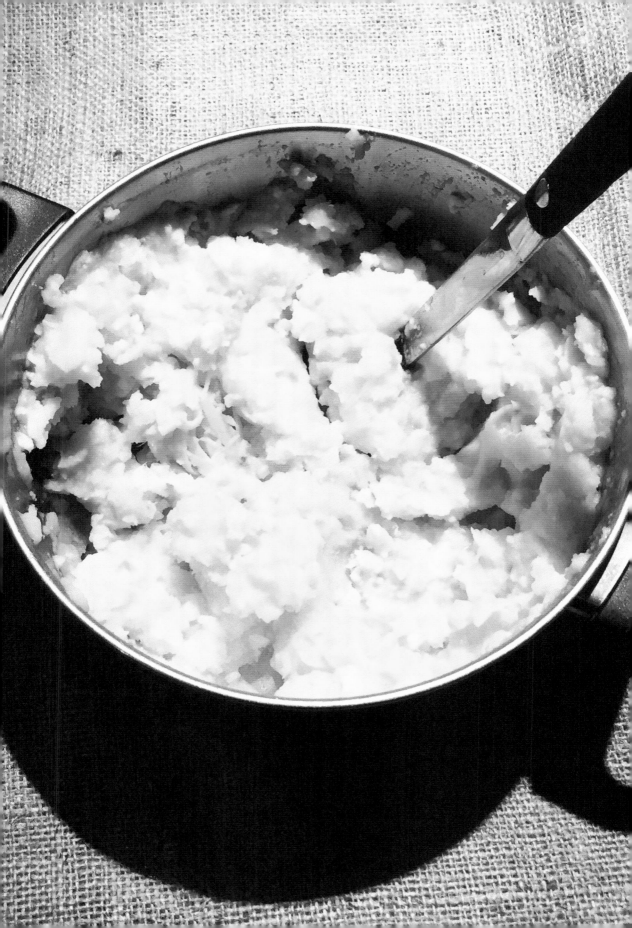

Roasted Aubergine & Courgette

This is a great one for BLW beginners and very easy to make – I love meals that I can quickly prepare and pop into the oven.

- -

Prep Time: 10 mins
Cook Time: 30 mins
Yields: 4

- -

Ingredients

1 courgette
1 aubergine
Olive oil
2 tbsp oregano

- -

Method

- Heat oven to 180°C
- Slice both courgette and aubergine into rounds and place onto baking trays
- Drizzle with olive oil and sprinkle with oregano
- Place in the oven and bake for 30-40 minutes until tender.

Side dishes

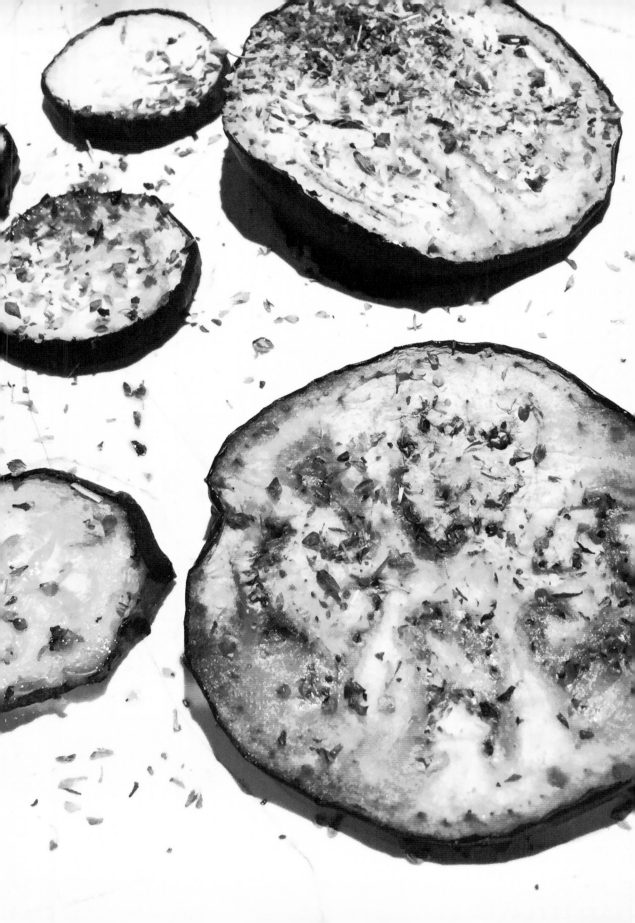

Crispy Parsnip Fries

Prep Time: 5 mins
Cook Time: 40 mins
Yields: 3-4

Ingredients

5 parsnips, peeled and cut into skinny fries
Olive oil for drizzling
1 tbsp dried rosemary
1 tbsp dried oregano

Method

- Heat oven to 180°C
- Simply place parsnips on a roasting tray, drizzle with olive oil and sprinkle with herbs
- Place in the oven for 30-40 minutes until soft on the inside and slightly golden and crisp on the outside

Side dishes

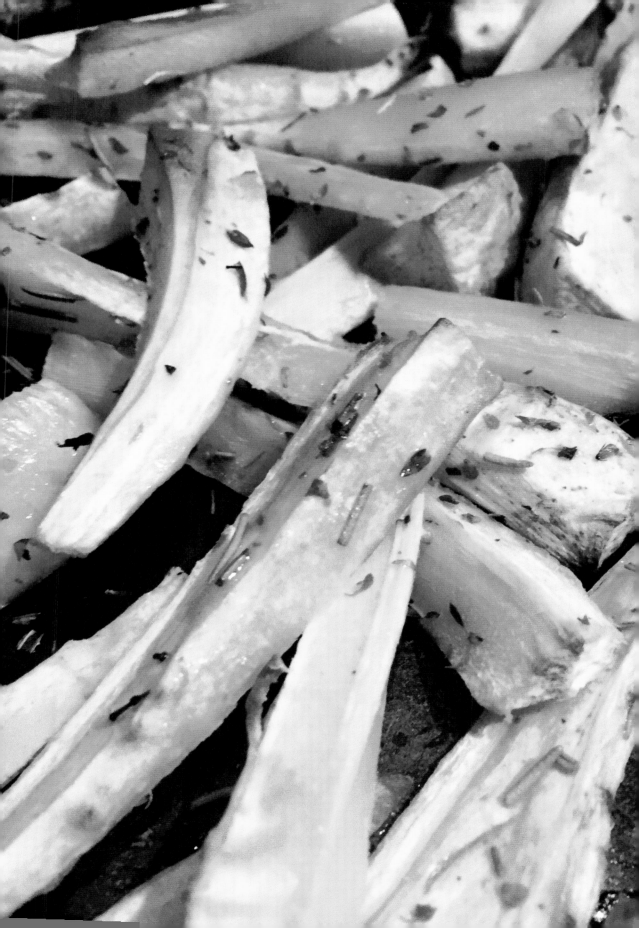

Carrot Fries

Seeing as we now have courgette and carrot etc. as subs of pasta why not carrot for chips?! Annabelle loves the sweetness of carrots and the finger shape of these make them ideal for BLW beginners too.

- -

Prep Time: 5 mins
Cook Time: 35 mins
Yields: 2

- -

Ingredients

4 carrots, peeled and chopped slightly larger than french fries
Dried oregano
Dried rosemary
Olive oil

- -

Method

- ■ Heat oven to 190°C
- ■ Parboil the carrots for 5 minutes
- ■ Drain and place onto a baking tray. Drizzle with olive oil and sprinkle with oregano and rosemary
- ■ Bake for 35-34 minutes until soft on the inside and crunchy on the outside

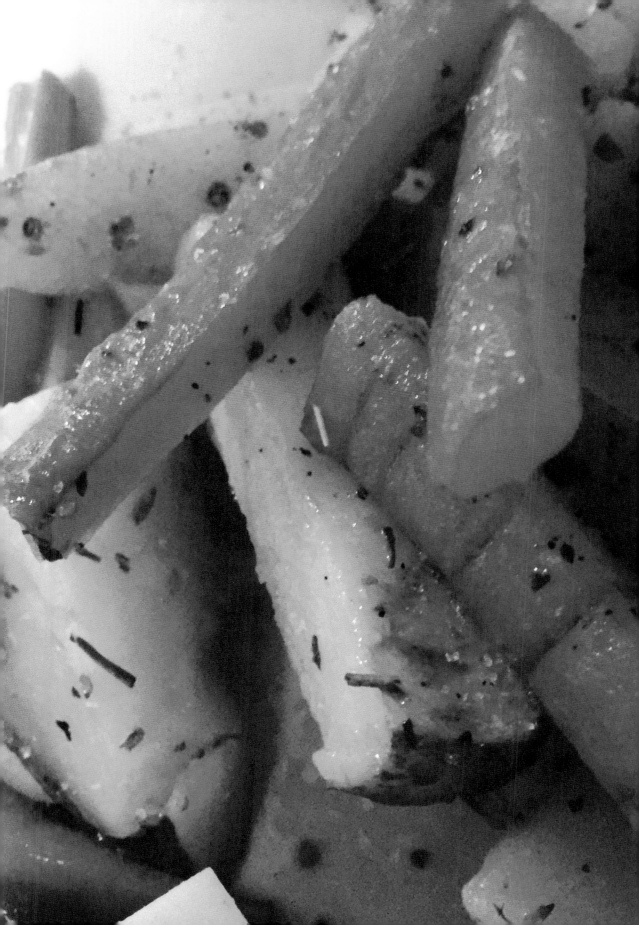

Sweet Potato Wedges

Excellent for BLW beginners! We enjoy these golden delights these with burgers, chilli, breaded chicken or simply on their own as a yummy, healthy snack.

- -

Prep Time: 5 mins
Cook Time: 35 mins
Yields: 2

- -

Ingredients

2 sweet potato wedges

- -

Method

- ■ Heat oven to 190°C
- ■ Cut sweet potatoes into wedges (half and then quarters)
- ■ Parboil for 5 minutes
- ■ Drain and then place onto a baking tray - drizzle sweet potatoes with olive oil and sprinkle with dried rosemary
- ■ Bake in the oven for 25 - 30 minutes - serve once cooled.

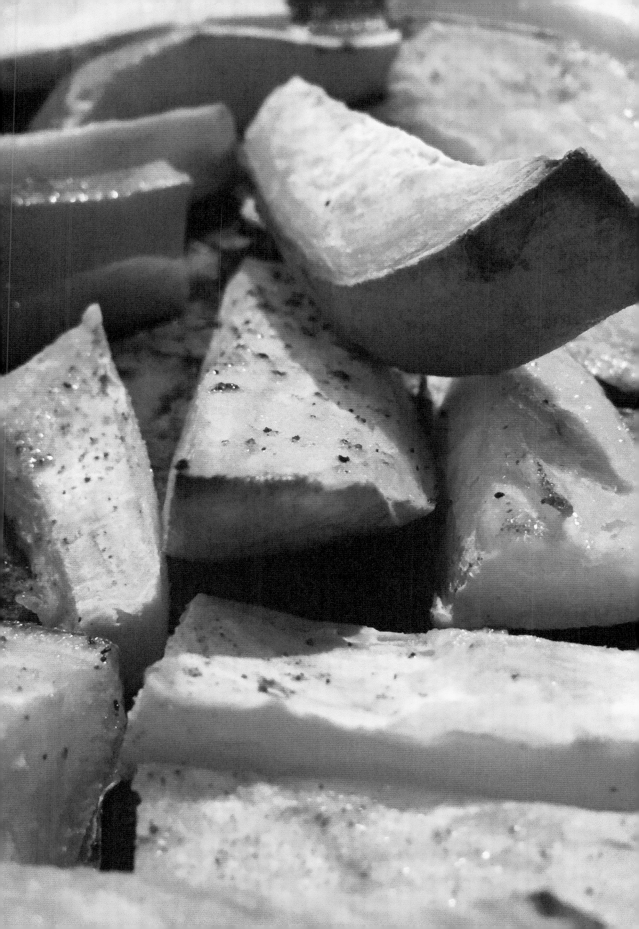

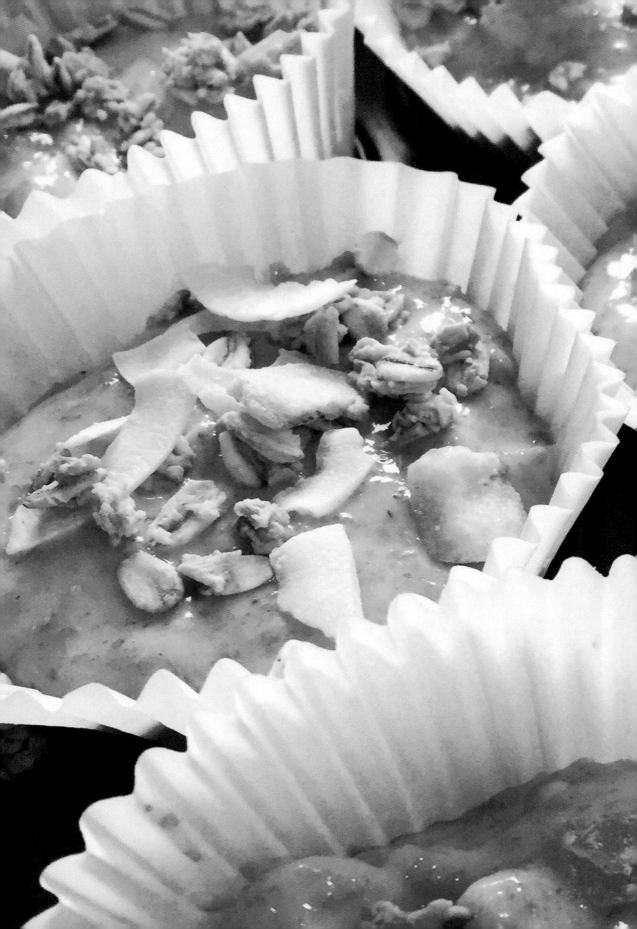

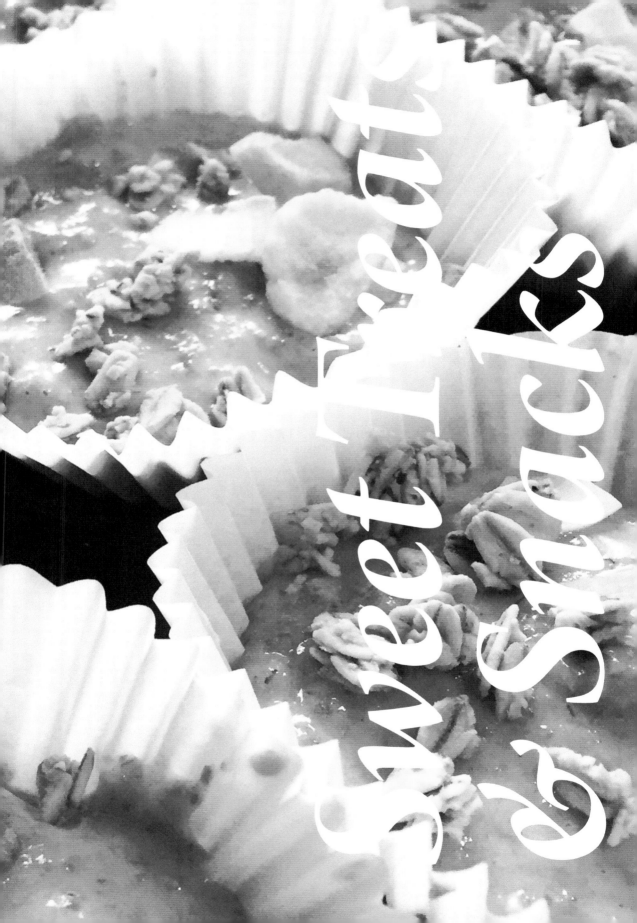

Sweet Treat & Snacks

No Bake
Peanut Butter Slice

This tasty peanut butter slice is so easy to whip together and makes a lovely treat for both you and your baby.

Prep Time: 10 mins
Cook Time: 0 mins
Yields: 10

Ingredients

1 1/2 cup peanut butter
1/2 cup maple syrup
1 cup oats

Method

■ Mix together peanut butter and maple syrup in a microwaveable bowl
■ Place peanut mix into the microwave for approx. 2 minutes until melted
■ Combine oats into the melted peanut mix - pour into a shallow dish
■ Place dish in the freezer for 1 hour and then transfer to the fridge

Sweet Treats & Snacks

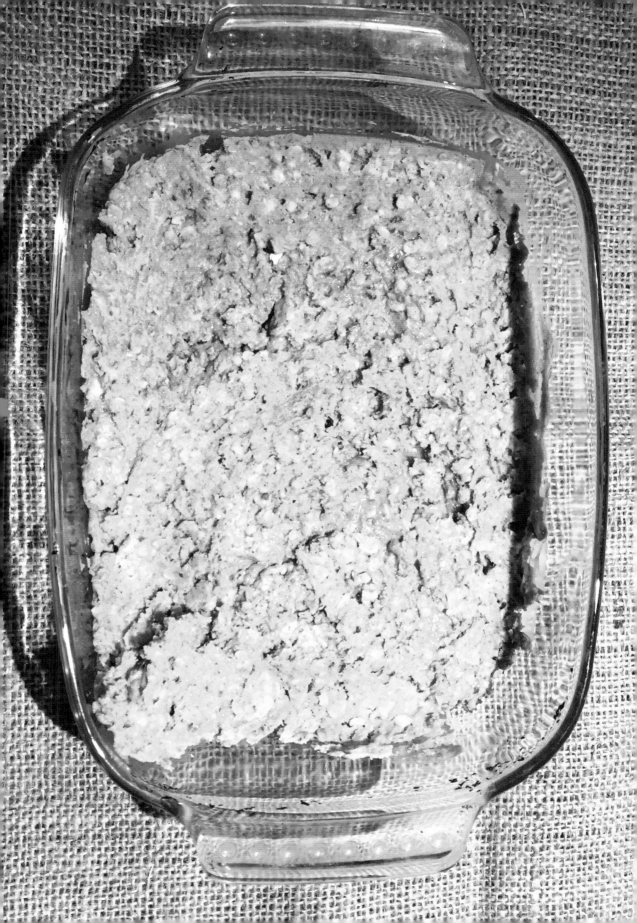

Strawberry, Blueberry & White Chocolate Muffins

These really are a treat with the white chocolate addition, however they are made with wholemeal flour so if you omit the white chocolate they are actually very healthy and would make a delicious breakfast muffin.

Prep Time: 10 mins
Cook Time: 25 mins
Yields: 12

Ingredients

¾ cup (180ml) vegetable oil
1 cup thick natural full fat yoghurt (or soya for CMA)
1/3 cup maple or agave syrup
2 cups wholemeal plain flour
2 teaspoons baking powder
1 teaspoon cinnamon, ground
2 eggs
1/2 cup blueberries (fresh or frozen)
1/2 cup strawberries, diced
1/3 cup white choc chips (optional)
3/4 cup crunchy granola, plus extra to sprinkle a top each muffin

Method

- Heat oven to 180°C
- Combine oil, eggs, yoghurt and maple syrup in a large bowl
- Add flour, baking powder and cinnamon and stir to combine
- Add blueberries, strawberries, white choc chips and granola and gently fold to combine.
- Pour the mixture into 12 muffin cases and bake for 15-25 mins - until golden and cooked through

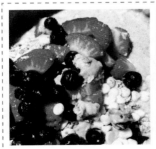 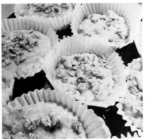 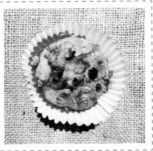

Sweet Treats & Snacks

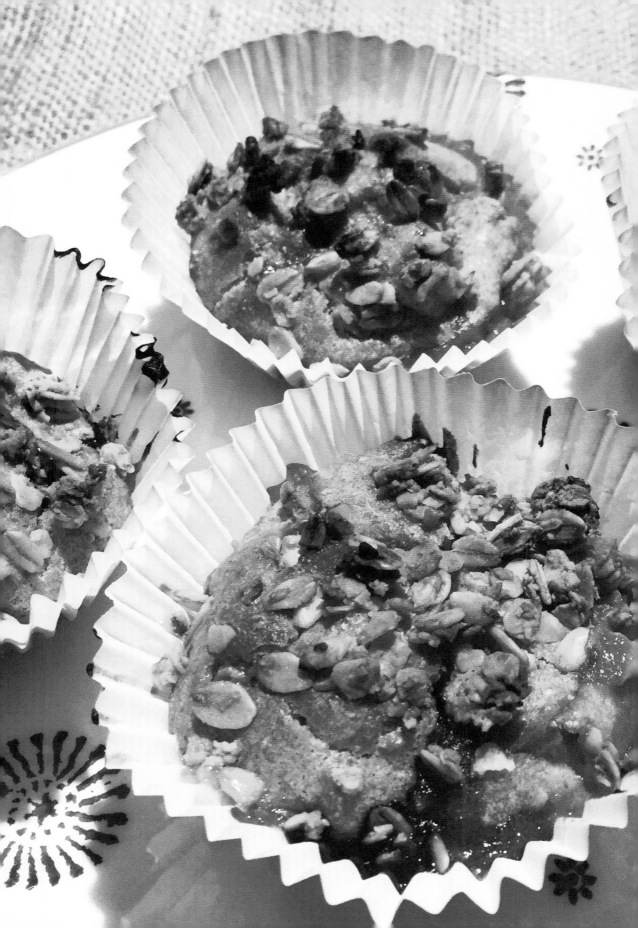

Blueberry & Strawberry Banana Bread

This is super healthy and naturally sweet loaf is ideal for a sweet toothed baby or mummy in need of a guilt free treat! Enjoy this wonderful loaf for breakfast, lunch or as a mid morning or afternoon snack. The granola on top is optional and best avoided if you don't want to use any refined sugar.

Prep Time: 15 mins
Cook Time: 45 mins
Yields: 1 loaf

Ingredients

2 cups (240g) whole wheat flour
1 tsp baking powder
½ tsp baking soda
1 tbsp (14g) unsalted butter, melted
1 egg
1 ½ tsp vanilla extract or paste
2 bananas, mashed
¼ cup (60g) plain full fat yogurt
3 tbsp (45ml) maple syrup
¼ cup (60ml) full fat milk
½ cup (80g) diced fresh strawberries (about 4 medium-large)
½ cup (70g) fresh or frozen blueberries
½ cup granola to sprinkle on top (optional)

Method

- Heat oven to 180°C and line a 9"x5" loaf pan
- In a small bowl, whisk together the flour, baking powder and baking soda
- In a separate bowl, whisk together the butter, egg, milk and vanilla. Stir in the mashed banana, yogurt, and maple syrup
- Slowly add wet ingredients to dry until you achieve a smooth batter
- Pour mix into a lined loaf tin and sprinkle with granola for added crunch (optional)
- Bake for 40-50 minutes, or until golden and cooked through

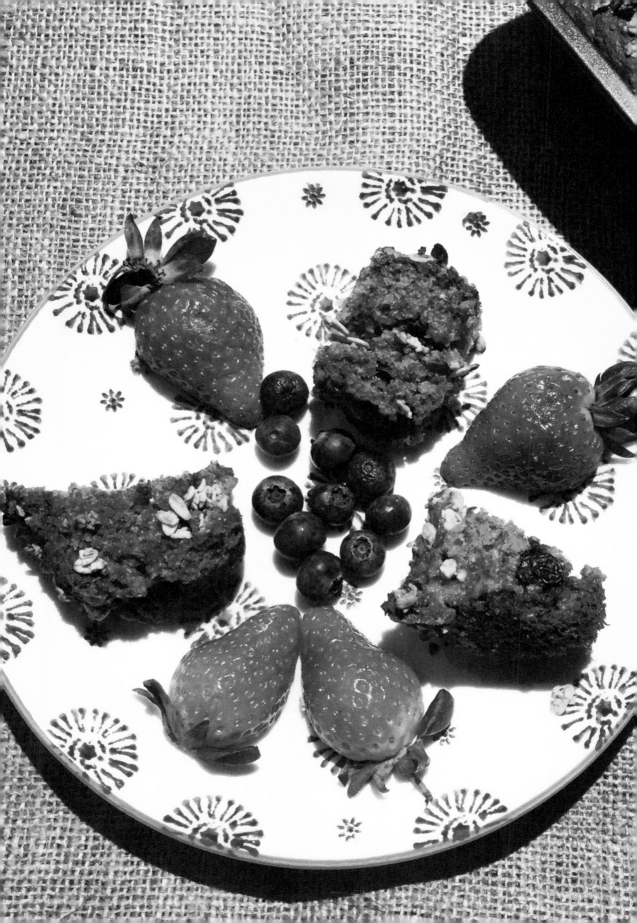

Mixed Berry & Oat Loaf

Prep Time: 15 mins
Cook Time: 50 mins
Yields: 4

Ingredients

2 cups self raising flour
1 tsp cinnamon
1/2 cup agave or maple syrup (I used agave)
3/4 cup veg oil
2 eggs
1 cup thick natural yoghurt (or plain soya for cows milk allergy)
1 tsp vanilla bean paste or extract
1 1/2 cup of frozen mixed berries
1/4 cup old fashioned oats (the cheap ones, not instant)
OR oats if you want to go completely sugar free
1/2 cup granola to sprinkle on top before baking

Method

- Heat oven to 180°C
- In a large bowl mix flour, cinnamon and oats
- In a separate bowl or jug mix agave, oil, eggs, yogurt and vanilla
- Slowly pour the wet ingredients into dry and whisk to create a lovely smooth thick batter
- Gentle fold through the frozen mixed berries
- Pour the mix into a lined loaf tin and sprinkle with granola (you could use oats, there healthier but not as tasty)
- Bake for 45-50 minutes until slightly golden and cooked through

Additional Info

This would be amazing with some white or milk choc chips for a naughtier treat! Note this is a moist cake due to the mixed berries but I find this helps Annabelle eat it - she just gags on dry cakes.

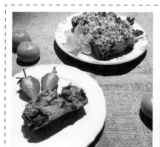
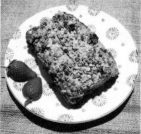
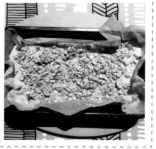

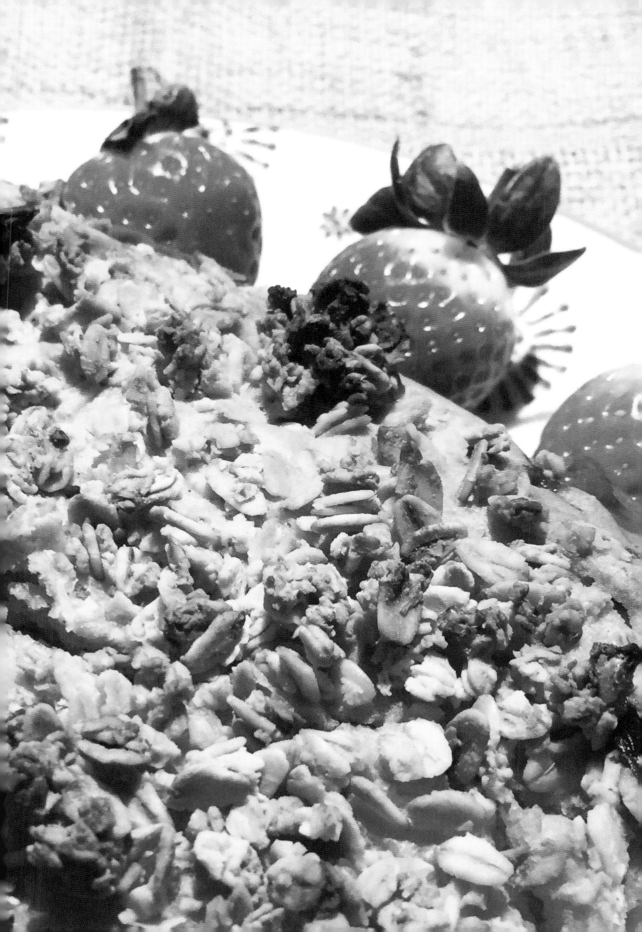

Peanut Butter Swirl Brownies

Prep Time: 15 mins
Cook Time: 30 mins
Yields: 12

Ingredients

1 egg
1/2 cup old fashioned oats
3/4 cup smooth peanut butter (I recommend the Whole Earth brand as its 97% peanuts)
1 tsp baking powder
1/2 cup coco powder
1/2 cup maple syrup
1/4 cup semi skimmed milk or soya for cows milk allergy
6oz vanilla Greek yogurt (or soya)

Method

- Heat oven to 180°C
- Simply blitz all ingredients except the peanut butter in a food processor
- Pour into a lined oven dish
- Pop peanut butter in the microwave for 30 seconds until melted and drizzle over the brownie batter
- Use a knife to mix peanut butter into swirls across the batter mix - it doesn't need to be perfect
- Bake in the oven for 20-25 minutes. Leave to cool and then place in the fridge for at least two hours before serving.

Additional Info

Some nuts and white chocolate chips in the brownie mix would make this recipe even more amazing!

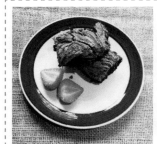
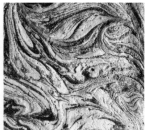
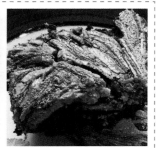

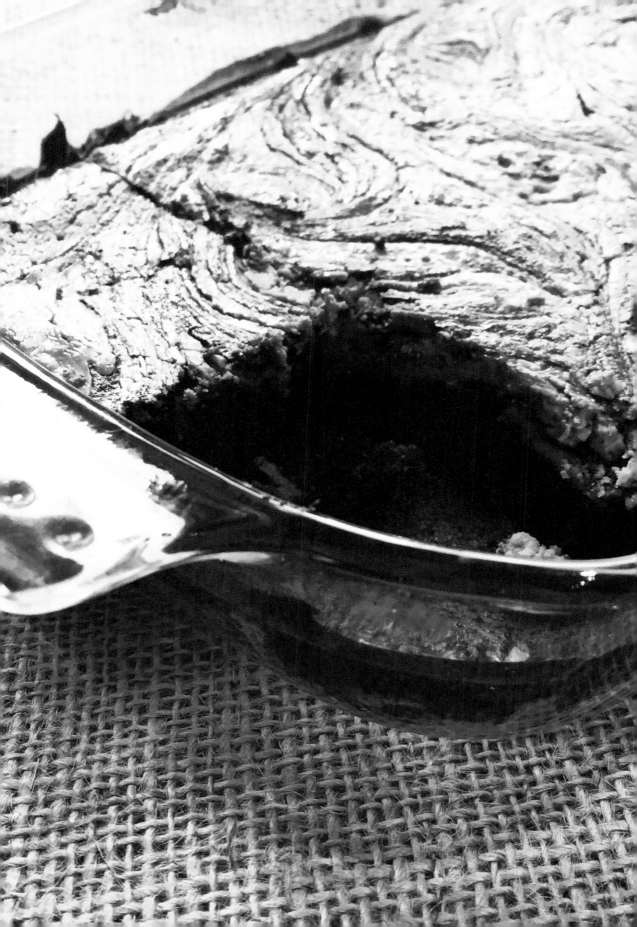

Tropical Peach Muffins

Prep Time: 15 mins
Cook Time: 30 mins
Yields: 12

Ingredients

3/4 cup vegetable oil
2 eggs
1 cup vanilla yogurt
1/3 cup agave syrup
2 cups wholemeal flour
2 tsp baking powder
1 tsp cinnamon
1 cup of peaches, peeled and cut in 1cm square chunks
3/4 cup tropical granola plus extra for the top

Method

- Heat oven to 180°C
- Mix eggs, yogurt, agave and oil in a large bowl
- Sift in the flour, cinnamon and baking powder - whisk to combine
- Gently stir in the peaches and granola
- Divide between 12 muffin cases - sprinkle with extra tropical granola
- Bake for 20-25 minutes or until cooked through

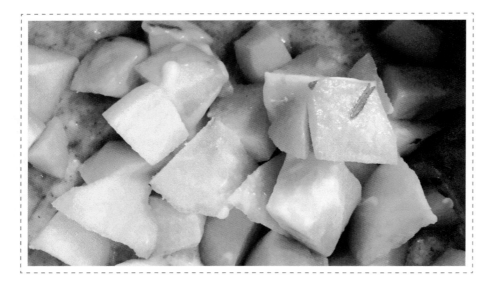

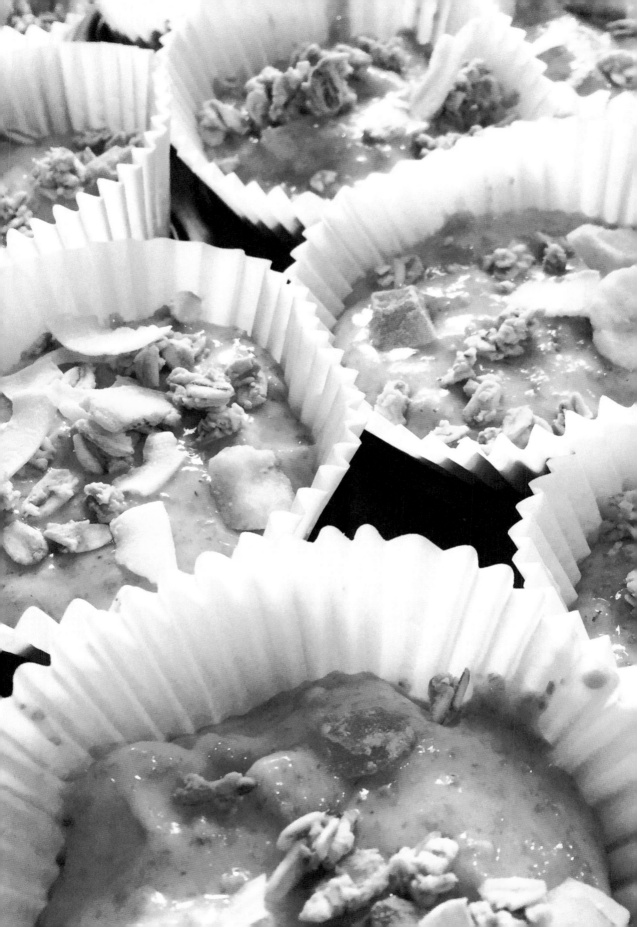

Mixed Berry Muffins

These are the best muffins I've made to date, I think using vanilla yogurt instead of plain and frozen berries instead of fresh have really upped the moisture. I really had to stop myself from eating the whole lot and had to remind myself that they were for Annabelle… naughty mummy!

- -

Prep Time: 15 mins
Cook Time: 30 mins
Yields: 12

- -

Ingredients

2 1/2 cups plain flour
2 1/2 tsp baking powder
3/4 cup brown sugar
2 eggs
3/4 cup vanilla yogurt (soya for cows milks allergy)
3/4 cup vegetable oil
1 1/2 cup frozen mixed berries
1/2 cup plain granola to sprinkle on top

- -

Method

- Preheat your oven to 180°C
- Mix eggs, yogurt and oil in a large bowl
- Sift in the flour, baking powder and brown sugar - mix to combine
- Gently fold in the mixed berries
- Divide between 12 muffin cases
- Sprinkle granola on top - place in the oven and bake for 15 - 20 minutes or until cooked through

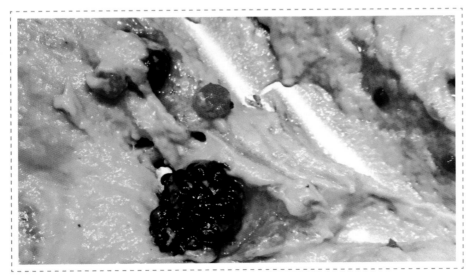

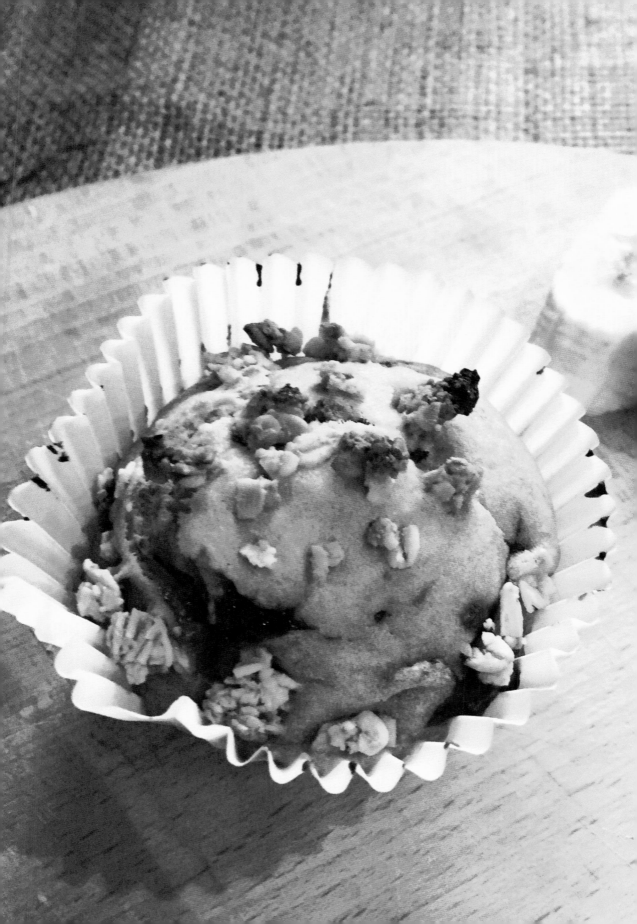

Peanut Butter Bites

Prep Time: 5 mins
Cook Time: 0 mins
Yields: 2

- -

Ingredients

2/3 cup peanut butter
1/3 cup milk (almond or coconut works best but soya or cows will work fine)
1/4 cup old fashioned oats (not instant)

- -

Method

- ■ Combine peanut butter and milk in the microwave for two minutes and then stir to combine
- ■ Mix in the oats
- ■ Wait for the mix to cool and then shape into bite size pieces, once shaped pop them in the fridge for 15 minutes
- ■ Excellent served with fruit and cheese

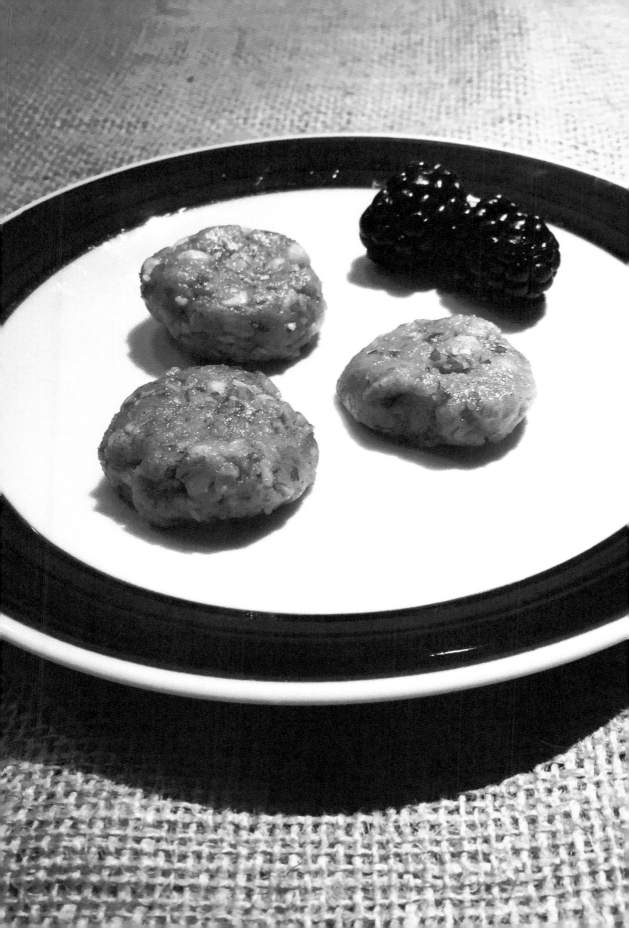

Ferrero Rocher Yogurt

Prep Time: 2 mins
Cook Time: 0 mins
Yields: 1

Ingredients

1 tsp Nutella
2 tbsp yogurt (soya for cows milk allergy)
1 tbsp old fashioned oats (not instant)

Method

■ Simply mix the ingredients into a bowl and enjoy!

Sweet Treats & Snacks

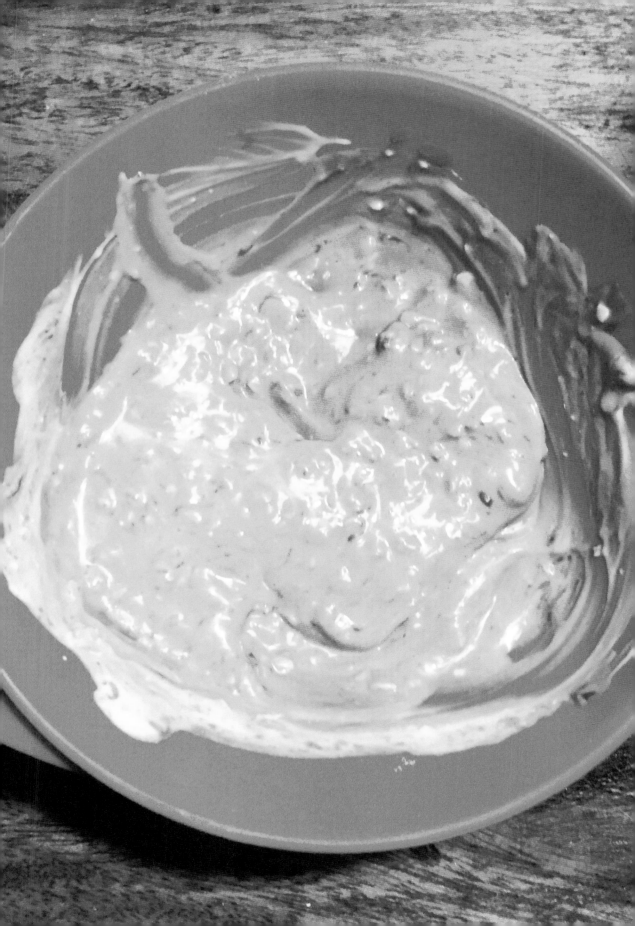

Strawberry Scones

Prep Time: 15 mins
Cook Time: 25 mins

- -

Ingredients

2 cups ground almonds
1 1/2 cups plain flour
2 eggs
1/4 cup veg oil
1 tbs agave or maple syrup
1 tsp vanilla bean paste
1 cup strawberries, diced
50ml milk (soya for cows milk allergy)

- -

Method

- Heat oven to 180°C
- Simply mix all of the ingredients together in a large bowl to form a dough/ or use a food processor
- Fold through the strawberries mushing them well into the dough - the mushier the better!
- Roll out the dough to a 2cm thickness and cut into rounds using a scone cutter
- Place scones onto a lined baking tray and bake for 20-25 minutes

Sweet Treats & Snacks

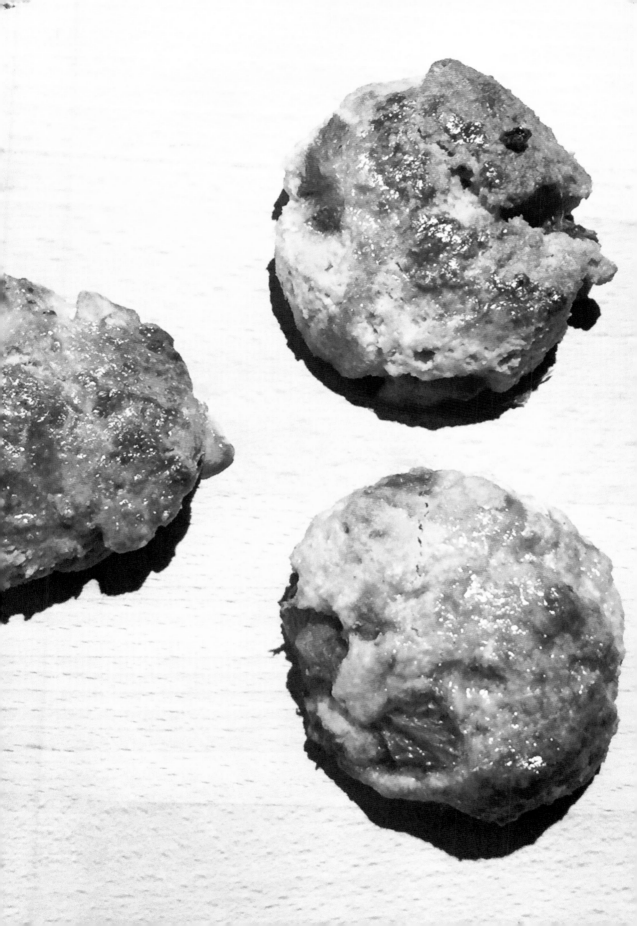

Peanut Butter Banana

Prep Time: 3 mins
Yields: 1

- -

Ingredients

1 banana
Dollops of peanut butter

- -

Method

- Simply peel a banana and then cut it into quarters - for older babies with good pincer grip they may prefer round 1cm slices
- Spread the peanut butter on top of the banana slices and serve - so simple!

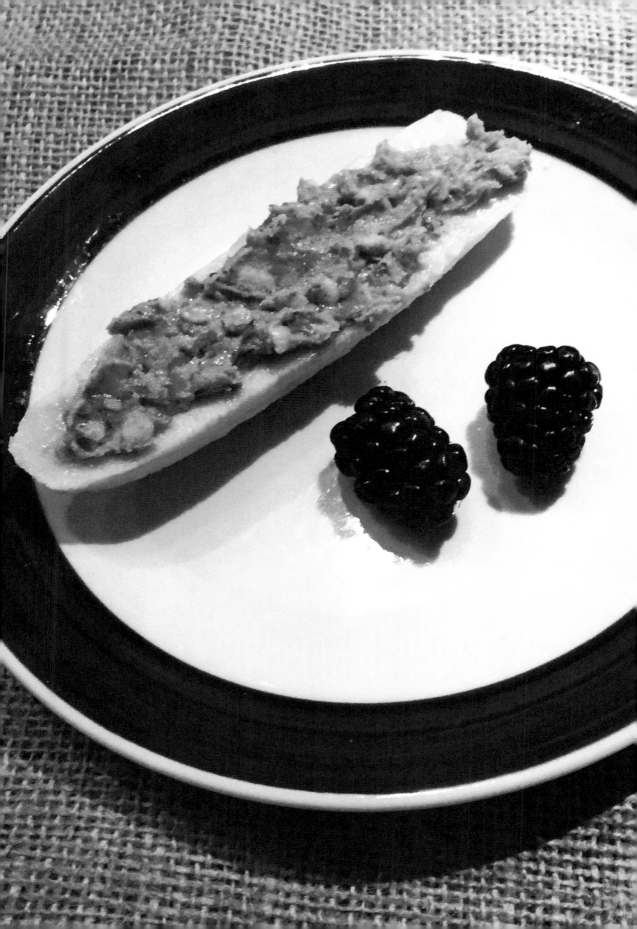

Strawberry Coconut Loaf

Prep Time: 15 mins
Cook Time: 35 mins
Yields: 8

- -

Ingredients

1/2 cup coconut flour
½ cup brown sugar
2 teaspoons baking powder
¾ cup vegetable oil
2 eggs
1 cup thick natural yoghurt (or plain soya for cows milk allergy)
1 teaspoon vanilla paste
1 cups of strawberries, quartered

- -

Method

- Heat oven to 180°C
- Sift flour, baking powder and sugar into a large bowl - mix well
- Add eggs, oil, vanilla and yogurt - whisk well to combine
- Gently stir in the strawberries
- Pour mix into a lined loaf tin
- Bake for 35 - 45 minutes - checking often

Sweet Treats & Snacks

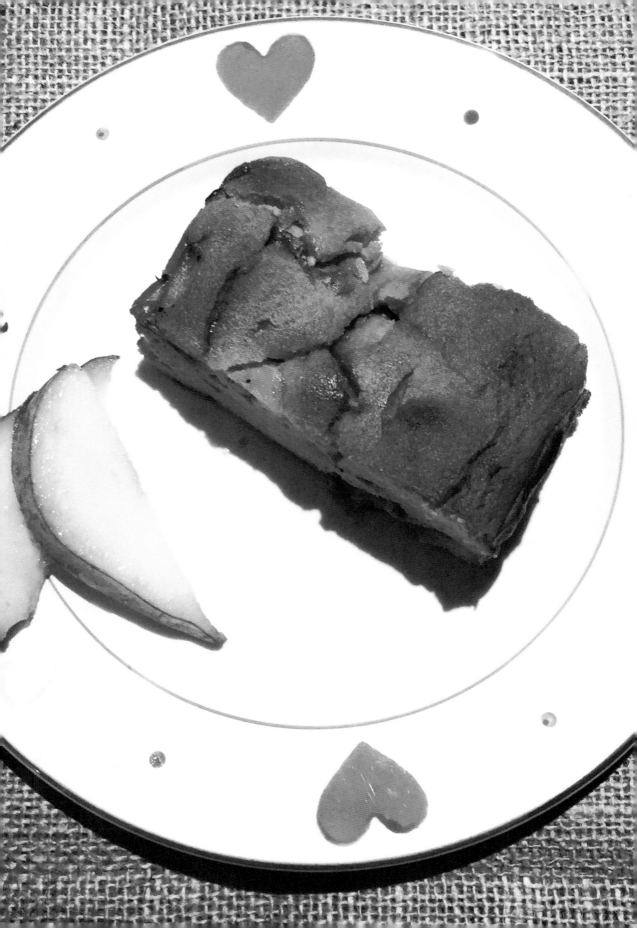

Baked Pears with Cinnamon

Prep Time: 10 mins
Cook Time: 50 mins
Yields: 4

- -

Ingredients

4 pears, peeled and cut into 4 - ensure seeds are removed
2 tbsp brown sugar
1/2 cup apple juice

- -

Method

- Heat oven to 180°C
- Simple placed your chopped pears into an ovenproof dish
- Pour the apple juice over the pears - use a spoon to splash juice over pears to ensure they have all been coated (this will stop them turning brown)
- Sprinkle the brown sugar evenly on top
- Place into the oven and bake for 50 minutes until soft

Sweet Treats & Snacks

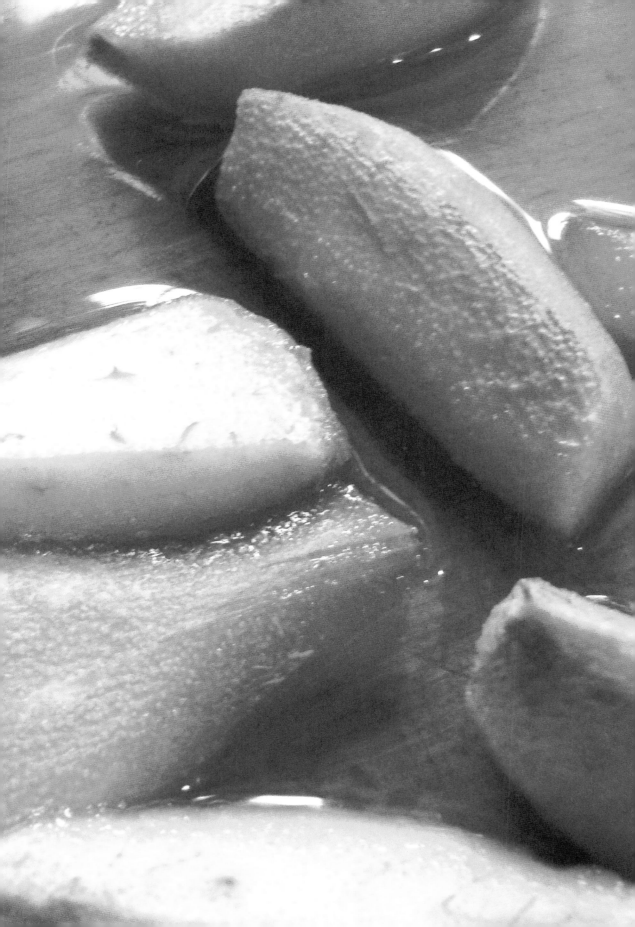

Healthy Prune Cookies

Prep Time: 15 mins
Cook Time: 20 mins
Yields: 10

Ingredients

3 bananas OR (400g) banana puree
4 tbsp butter (use soya or almond butter for cows milk allergy)
1 tbsp vegetable oil
4 tbsp agave syrup
1 1/2 cups oats
4 dried prunes, finely chopped

Method

- Heat oven to 180°C
- Mush bananas in a bowl with a fork until smooth
- Mix butter, oil and agave syrup in with the mashed banana then stir in the oats and chopped prunes.
- Using your hands shape heaped tablespoon quantities into 10 cookies and place onto a lined baking tray
- Bake cookies for 20 minutes or until then turn golden brown

Sweet Treats & Snacks

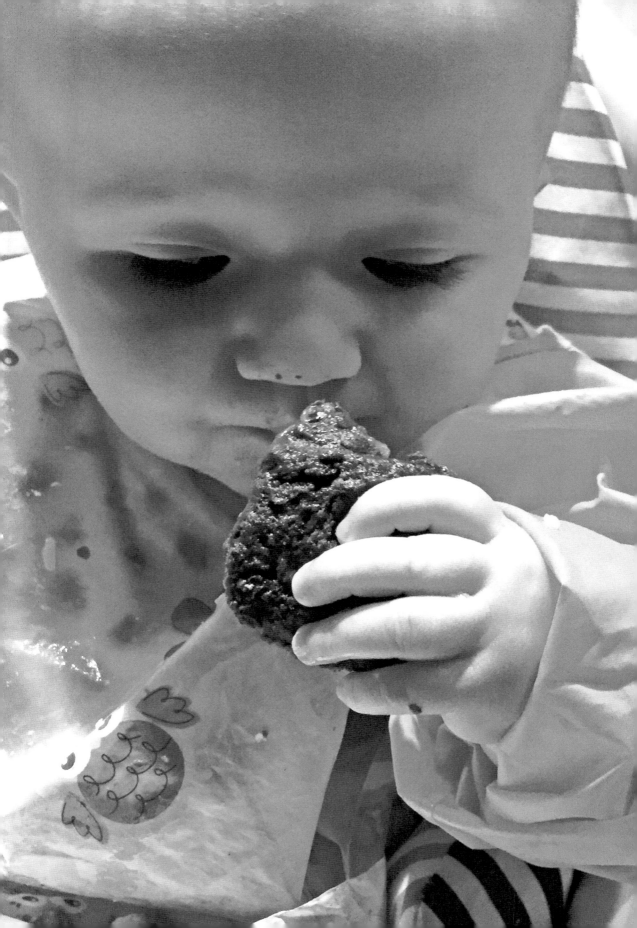

Wholemeal Blueberry Muffins

Prep Time: 10 mins
Cook Time: 20 mins
Yields: 12

Ingredients

¾ cup vegetable oil
2 eggs
1 cup thick natural yoghurt (use soya for cows milk allergy)
1/3 cup agave syrup
2 cups wholemeal flour
2 teaspoons baking powder
1 teaspoon ground cinnamon
1 cup blueberries
3/4 cup old fashioned oats

Method

- Heat oven to 190°C
- Line a muffin tray with 12 cases
- Combine eggs, oil, yoghurt and agave syrup in a large bowl - mix well
- Add dry ingredients (flour, baking powder and cinnamon) to wet and mix well
- Stir in the blueberries and oats
- Spoon mix between 12 muffin cases
- Bake for 15-20 minutes until slightly golden and cooked through

Sweet Treats & Snacks

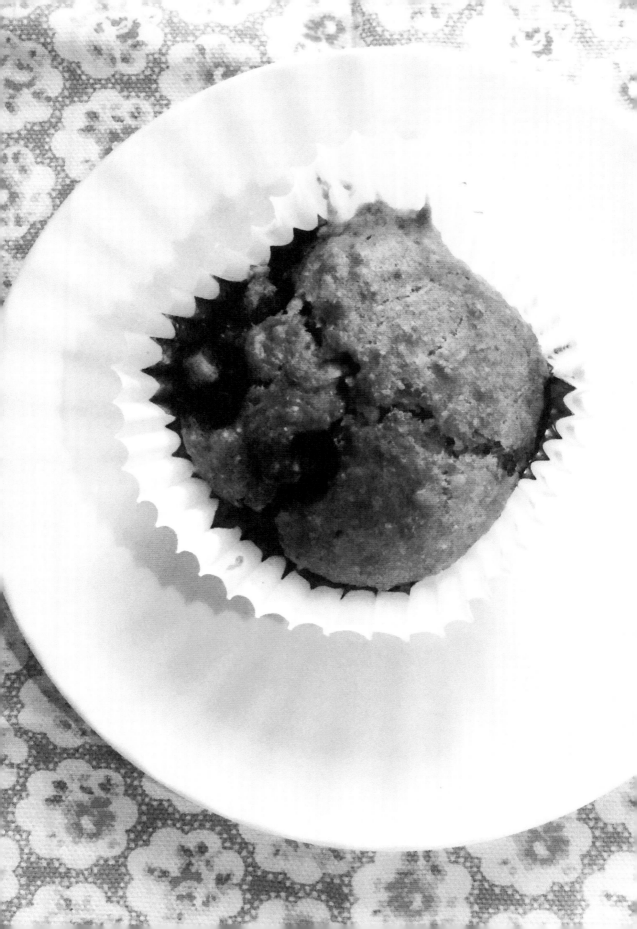

Mum and Baby Meal Plan

Monday
Breakfast: Thick porridge with maple syrup and blueberries
Lunch: Ham and cheese toasty
Dinner: Shepherds pie

Tuesday
Breakfast: Blueberry muffins
Lunch: Cheese and apple tortilla and choice of fruit
Dinner: Jacket potato with tuna (mixed with sweetcorn and natural full fat yogurt)

Wednesday
Breakfast: Toast fingers and choice of fruit
Lunch: Tuna and cheese melt
Dinner: Meatballs and penne pasta

Thursday
Breakfast: Thick porridge with maple syrup and strawberries
Lunch: Scrambled egg on toast with sliced cherry tomatoes and cheese slices
Dinner: Turkey pasta bake

Friday
Breakfast: Fried egg on toast with pear slices
Lunch: Turkey and cranberry sandwich & choice of fruit
Dinner: Burgers and sweet potato fries with salad

Saturday:
Breakfast: Eggy bread with choice of fruit
Lunch: Avocado on toast/ sliced banana and cheese
Dinner: Chicken Rosti

Sunday:
Breakfast: Scotch pancakes with nutella topped with banana or mixed berries
Lunch: Pate on toast & baked pear with cinnamon
Dinner: Chicken bake

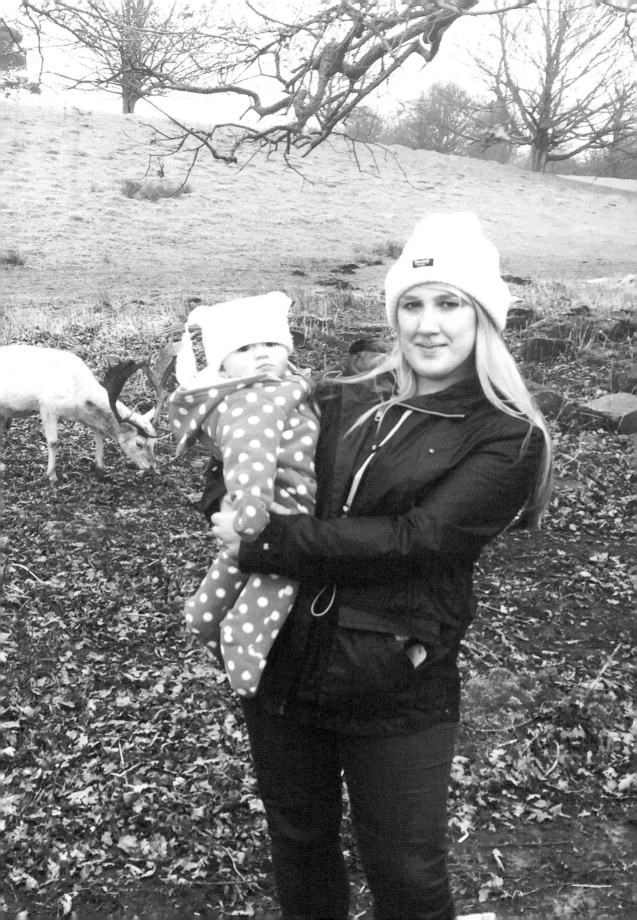

Beginners 4 week plan

Week 1:

Steamed carrot sticks
Steamed broccoli
Steamed cauliflower
Mashed potato made with unsalted butter – give to baby on
a loaded spoon.
Sweet potato wedges
Steamed celery sticks
Roasted aubergine sticks

Week 2:

Roasted courgette sticks
Green beans
Mashed butternut squash – given to baby on a loaded spoon
Mashed potato served on a loaded spoon with steamed carrot sticks
Mushed peas served on a loaded spoon with steamed cauliflower and
broccoli
Steamed celery sticks with steamed apple
Steamed carrot sticks with toast and steamed apple

Week 3:

Mashed potato with green beans and over ripe pear
Toast with melted cheese and steamed apple sprinkled with cinnamon
Sweet potato wedges and mango slices
Toast soldiers, sticks of mild cheese and steamed apples
Bread topped with grated apple and sprinkled with cheese – grilled until
melted – served in sticks
Sweet potato wedges, roasted courgette and cooked fusilli pasta with
grated cheese
Eggy bread sprinkled with cinnamon

Week 4:

Mushed banana served on a loaded spoon with steamed celery sticks and
cauliflower
Strips of chicken, cheese sticks and overripe pear
Roasted sweet red pepper, courgette and aubergine.
Plain yogurt mixed with fruit puree – served loaded onto a spoon
Mashed avocado on toast
Strips of beef, mashed butternut squash and steamed apple
Mango slices, mashed banana on toasted, cheese sticks

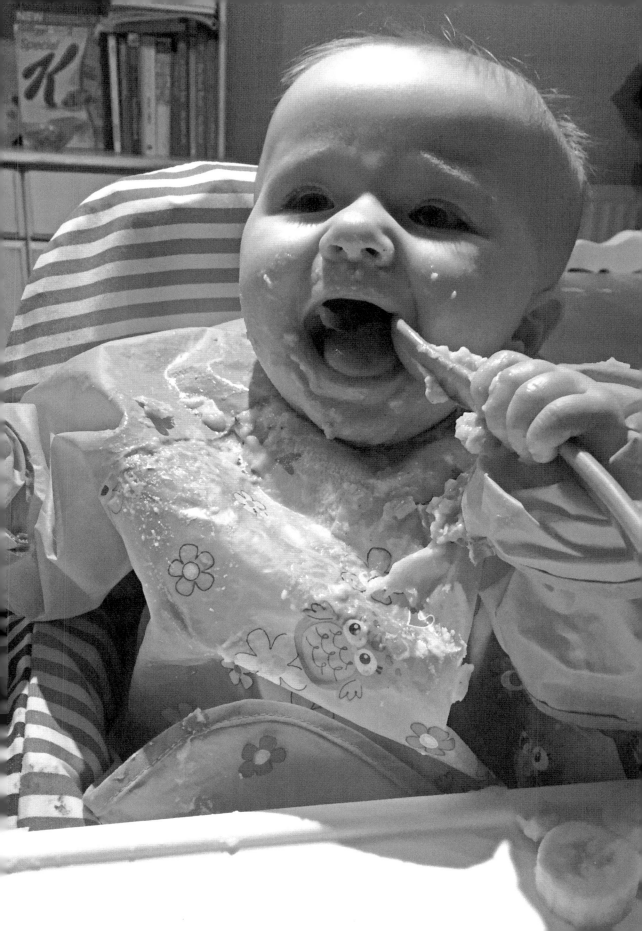

BLW Tips:

- Buy frozen veg and cook in microwave – this saves time and money!

- Fruit can be cooked in the microwave too

- Always have pears in the house – they are a super easy go to!

- Your baby wont actually eat anything to begin with and that's fine – at the start it's all about baby exploring different tastes and textures

- Invest in an overall bib with sleeves – put baby it in from day one so they get use to it

- The overall will be too big to start with so ensure baby has a bib on underneath

- Put baby in highchair a month before you start to get him/her use to it

- Starting in a Bumbo seat is fine

- Invest in surface wipes

- Invest in a splash mat

- Be prepared for mess but try to see it as your baby having messy play time every day

- Always have baby wipes to hand

- Don't stress

- Cook food when baby is asleep so your not in a mad dash

- Don't feed baby at set times, feed him/her when it suits you in the day – this can be at different times every day to start with

- Try to feed baby in-between milk feeds or just after so they are not hungry

- Don't try baby with solids if they are tired

- Don't give your baby honey – use maple syrup instead

- Don't feed your baby fromage frais as they have more sugar than a chocolate bar!

- Try to find a local NCT weaning course they cost about £30 and are a great help